S I M P L E

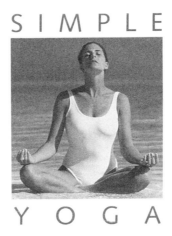

Y O G A

Cybèle Tomlinson

Foreword by Vimala McClure

CONARI PRESS
Berkeley, California

Conari Press books are distributed by Publishers Group West.

Cover Photograph © Nancy Brown/ImageBank
Cover and book design: Claudia Smelser
Interior Photographs © 1999 Philip Kakke

Library of Congress Cataloging-in-Publication Data

Tomlinson, Cybèle.
  Simple yoga / Cybèle Tomlinson
    p cm .— (Simple wisdon book)
  ISBN: 1–57324–195–4
    1. Yoga, Haòha—Therapeutic use. I. Title. II. Series.
  RM 727.Y64 T66 2000
  613.7'046—dc21   00–020680

Printed in the United States of America on recycled paper.

00 01 02 RRD(NW) 10 9 8 7 6 5 4 3 2 1

This book is dedicated to my grandmothers,

Eleanor Kingsley Lawford
and *Berenis Fleming Tomlinson.*

SIMPLE YOGA

Foreword ix

Introduction 1

one What Is Yoga? 3

two The Roots of Yoga 17

three The Yoga Path 29

four Principles of Yoga Practice 49

five Finding a Yoga Class 71

six Yoga for Women 99

seven A Good Basic Routine 107

eight An Office Yoga Routine 135

To Learn More 141

Acknowledgments 145

Index 147

FOREWORD

by Vimala McClure
author of *A Woman's Guide to Tantra Yoga*

Yoga, a great body of wisdom from the East, made its way West as early as the mid-1800s, when the great Swami Vivekananda brought his system of Raja Yoga, which was based on the ancient sage Patanjali's eightfold path, from India to the United States and Great Britain. Since then Westerners have had a keen interest in yoga and all its practices, philosophies, and ethical principles. There are many different kinds of yoga, and in this book Cybèle Tomlinson simply and effortlessly describes some of them, from ancient systems to modern versions that have sprung up in the West. She answers a beginning student's questions in a way that is easily understood and is true to the tradition from which this great philosophy of life has originated.

I recommend this book as a wonderful starting point for anyone who is unfamiliar with yoga philosophy and practice and would like to try it. Cybèle has provided you with an ethical and philosophical framework and some postures that are perfect for a daily routine. You need seek no further; mastering the postures and the ideas behind them can easily form a yoga practice that you continue for life. I have found that "changing up" once in a while prevents boredom, and this book has helped refresh and revitalize my own practice. I use it, with my own book, in my yoga practice.

It is very refreshing to me to see that the author addresses issues of the disabled, the elderly, pregnant women, and children. The practice she describes here is not overly athletic, which is a great relief and something I also tried to achieve in my introductory book. I believe most people who want to start a yoga practice should begin with this simple routine, and continue with it for a long time before seeking anything more strenuous or complicated. The point of yoga postures is to put pressure on certain hormonal glands in the body to maintain hormonal balance and to keep the ligaments and muscles smooth, firm, and limber. All the postures in this book achieve these ends without overexerting the Western body, which is usually not accustomed to much stretching.

Cybèle also talks about the importance of breathing, which is such an everyday part of our lives that we often forget about it or neglect to recognize its importance as a vital tool for cleansing our bodies and minds, restoring vitality and peace, and calming anxiety. The postures shown in this book are complete and can help your body and mind stay in balance for years to come. Many of them have been part of my own yoga practice for more than twenty-seven years. It is a wonderful comfort to approach your everyday yoga practice not as a chore to be done, but as a gift you are receiving from the Great Creator. In this receptive mode, gratitude fills you as you slowly and carefully, with full concentration, move through each sequence of breathing, moving, and relaxing. You will always emerge from your session filled with the gift of life-giving energy circulating through your body and peace permeating your being.

I urge you to read this book and give it a try. Commit to it for a month and see what happens. You will probably find that you bring more calm energy to your work, you have less need for sleep, you begin gravitating toward foods that nourish you, and people around you begin noticing "something" different, and good, about you.

INTRODUCTION

This book is intended for people who are curious about yoga but don't know much about it. It is difficult to speak about yoga as any one thing: in fact, there are many different kinds of yoga, and they can vary quite widely in their approaches and their practices. But all yoga concerns itself with questions that have challenged human beings for a long time: How can we be truly, lastingly happy? How can we free ourselves fully from our suffering?

I have tried to present yoga in a simple way, giving you, the reader, a *feeling* for what yoga is—and for what it can be in your life. I've also briefly described the kinds of yoga that are most common in the West, in the hope that you will feel inspired to explore this rich tradition on your own.

one

WHAT IS YOGA?

The word *yoga* can conjure up an array of images: bodies twisting and contorting into impossible pretzel shapes, or long-haired Indian yogis sitting atop mountains, lost in a meditative trance. Some of us link yoga with hippies, and there is good reason for this association: yoga did, indeed, become more visible and popular in the '60s, when larger numbers of people—many of them young—in the West began to experiment with a variety of Eastern teachings.

Each of these associations paints part of the picture, but not all of it. Yoga can be—and often is—approached through the body, especially in the West. And there are many postures, some of which are quite challenging, that make up the physical aspect of yoga practice.

But yoga is much more than just physical exercise: it also embraces the realms of mind and spirit. At heart, yoga is more about a whole way of being, one that is not limited to mountaintop ascetics who choose to give up their worldly ties but is equally available to the busiest Westerner. In fact, many of the most influential yoga teachers of our day maintain families, which is hardly possible while living in a cave or on a mountain! And though yoga may have seemed for a time to be a "hippie thing," it has become increasingly mainstream, particularly since the early 1990s. It is an alive, evolving tradition that is evolving in ways that both reflect and respond to the needs of people living in the twenty-first century.

The Sanskrit word *yoga* has multiple meanings. Its root, *yuj*, can be translated as "to yoke," "to fasten," or "to harness." Yoga is most commonly translated simply as "union," though it can also mean "discipline." It's often spoken of as the discipline, or process, of uniting mind, body, and spirit.

The origins of yoga are in India. It is believed to have existed in some form for as long as 5,000 years—and possibly longer. Over time, yoga has branched off into a multitude of schools, making it a very rich and complex tradition with many different approaches and techniques. Enormous scholarly effort has gone into sorting out these various forms and understanding their differences.

What can be said about all forms of yoga, though, whatever their approach and methodology, is that their goals are the same. The real aim of yoga is to liberate human beings from suffering and bring us to a place of deep, lasting peace and limitless happiness. One of the contemporary scholars of yoga, Georg Feuerstein, describes yoga as the "technology of ecstasy."

We all have moments of that joy—perhaps when we're skiing, listening to an exquisite piece of music, or thinking deeply about a complicated problem. Some people have felt these sorts of "highs" through hallucinogenic drugs. There is the feeling of complete immersion, total absorption; ordinary thinking is suspended. We're not aware of ourselves in the way we normally are; for a few seconds, or minutes, or maybe—if we're really lucky—a few hours, we forget who we are. But these are all fleeting experiences. Try as we might, we can't sustain this state: we can't will ourselves into it.

What would it be like to be this way all the time? Yoga tells us that not only is this possible, it is actually our natural state. It is our essential nature, our birthright. Through steady yoga practice we are given the means to reach this lasting joy.

In yoga, there are a number of terms for this essential nature—Self, Soul, *Atman, purusha,* the Absolute, the Supreme Spirit, the Universal Spirit, Ultimate Reality—and some people use the term God. The end goal of yoga is to fully *realize* our essential nature, or Self. Self-realization has nothing to do with thinking. It has nothing to do with language. It's completely beyond any sort of "normal" experience. Those who achieve this ecstatic state report that it's beyond description.

Another, more accessible way to think of the yoga is this: It's a means of bringing out and fully manifesting our highest, or greatest, potential. Yoga gives us capacities we did not have before—physical, mental, and spiritual. It shows us how to clear the path so that we can become more fully alive—more ourselves.

If you consider again those transitory moments of freedom

and peace that you have from time to time, these experiences are characterized by a feeling of *flow*. Everything around you seems to function harmoniously. And everything in yourself is likewise flowing smoothly toward the same end. Every part of you—body, mind, and heart—is engaged in and committed to whatever you're doing.

More commonly, though, we're not in this state of being wholly involved. We often experience discord or even opposition in ourselves. Consider how much of the time you are in some sort of mental debate about something. The subject can be important, because there's a big decision to be made, like whether or not to buy a new car. You want the car, but maybe you know that the money should be put toward your child's education. Or perhaps it's something as trivial as whether or not to pick up the phone when it rings. Or it can manifest just as general restlessness, a free-floating dissatisfaction with how things are in the moment: we want something, but we don't know exactly what, and so we don't know what to do with ourselves. When we experience states like this, we're fragmented. We're pulled in different directions and our energy can't be directed toward any one activity. This makes us feel stuck.

Yoga is about clearing away whatever is in us that prevents our living in the most full and whole way. With yoga, we become aware of how and where we are restricted—in body, mind, and heart—and how gradually to open and release these blockages. As these blockages are cleared, our energy is freed.

We start to feel more harmonious, more at one with ourselves. Our lives begin to flow—or *we* begin to flow more in our lives, regardless of the exterior circumstances.

WHO CAN DO YOGA?

Although yoga is fundamentally a spiritual path, it's a mistake to think that yoga practice requires a belief in God. Yoga is *not* a religion, though its history is interwoven with some of the major religions of India. Nor does a person's religion get in the way of yoga practice. Yoga is remarkably inclusive: there are yoga practitioners of all different religions as well as those who have no religious leanings whatsoever.

Yoga is open to anyone who is interested in it. Age is no barrier: you can start at any stage of life. And—contrary to what some people think—you don't have to be particularly flexible or strong in order to begin a yoga practice. There are no prerequisites to yoga except an open mind. The beauty of yoga is that it responds to the needs and interest of the individual. It can be used simply as a means to better health (and this is often what motivates people to try yoga in the first place) or it can be pursued with more passion as a whole way of life. Because of the tremendous variety within the world of yoga, anyone with sufficient curiosity and desire can find a suitable form that matches his or her nature.

The yoga that has become most popular in the West involves practice of physical postures (called *asanas*) and breathing techniques (called *pranayama*). These practices form the bulk of what is known as *Hatha* yoga—the yoga of force—which emphasizes strengthening and purifying the body. Hatha yoga is sometimes used as a general term to refer to the physicality of yoga practice, but it is also a complete system in and of itself.

In this branch of yoga, it is thought that in order to progress along the path toward self-realization, the mind and spirit must be contained in a healthy vessel. So Hatha Yoga begins with the body. (Traditionally, there are actually two previous stages to physical practice, which are called *yama*—guidelines governing our behavior toward others—and *niyama*—those that guide our behavior and attitudes toward ourselves. In the West, however, most people start with the physical practice.)

It makes sense to start with the body. Most of us feel better when we're physically well, and it's certainly more difficult to feel happy when we're unwell. Through the practice of postures and breath control, we approach the obstacles to our health. We clear the impurities that accumulate and lead to stagnation and disease. We work to restore and heal the body, making it function as optimally as possible. Once we are more healthy, we are in a better position to approach the other aspects of yoga practice.

Practice of the asanas—or postures—can impact us in fairly ob-vious ways. First of all, they make us more sensitive to our bod-ies; we become aware of where we're strong and where we're weak. We notice where we're flexible and where there's little or no movement. We notice how our physical freedom has been confined by our unconscious habits of holding and moving our-selves. As we work with the asanas, we build our strength and we identify and release the physical blockages that restrict our movements. The end result is that we improve posture, restore range of motion, and open up whole new possibilities for move-ment.

But yoga postures also operate in much subtler realms. The blood is cleansed and begins circulating in the body more effi-ciently, bringing more oxygen and nutrients to all the tissues. The internal organs are lightly massaged and stimulated, and the body's metabolism is increased and digestion improved. Even glandular activity can be affected by yoga. These effects can have a profound impact on how practitioners feel. After be-ginning yoga, many people report that they have more energy than before. In addition, because yoga is so calming to the ner-vous system, practitioners become more relaxed and at ease in their bodies.

Suppose your job requires that you sit a lot—either at a desk, in a car, or on a plane—and you notice that your back has been bothering you. Maybe you have even developed some chronic back pain. Through a few simple yoga postures you may be able to strengthen and mobilize your back so that you are able to sit for long periods without pain.

Or maybe your life has become very stressful and you have developed high blood pressure. Medical research has proven that relaxation, which is an essential part of yoga practice, can effectively relieve high blood pressure. In general, yoga is extremely useful for coping with stress—and stress, which affects all of us, is now being implicated as a major contributor to the development of many life-threatening diseases.

Yoga can be used to help with such diverse ailments as arthritis, asthma, or chronic fatigue; it can also prepare a woman to give birth, as well as to recover afterward. In fact, there are a huge number of health applications for yoga, and there are many people whose health has been significantly impacted by regular yoga practice. (Please be aware, however, that yoga is not meant to replace medical care and should be undertaken with the advice of a physician if you have a serious health problem.)

BEYOND THE BODY

As we practice yoga postures and breathing techniques, we continue to reap benefits. Often these improvements are most evident physically, at least in the beginning. Our bodies become more resilient and fluid. We can do more; we start feeling younger and more energetic. Our whole way of being in our bodies can change so dramatically that what was "normal" before is no longer acceptable: we have a new standard of health.

The mind can also be impacted by yoga practice. Many people report that their powers of concentration increase. People also find that memory is improved. In general, as yoga becomes more central to our lives, we become increasingly sensitive to the activity in our minds. We become aware of how much random mental movement there is most of the time. In particular, though, we notice our mental tendencies, or habits, and we begin to wake up to how these tendencies influence our actions.

Our mental patterns are revealed in the way that we practice yoga. For instance, sometimes our minds tell us—wrongly—that we are not capable of a particular posture. Or our minds can make us overly confident, pushing us beyond our proper limits. As we become aware of these automatic mental tendencies, we see how they can limit us, both on the yoga mat and in our daily lives. We begin to realize that our habits are essentially false beliefs we have about ourselves, and that, in fact, we are something more than what our minds may tell us. This dawning awareness of ourselves is supported in our yoga practice as we continue to observe and work with our habits. The practice of relaxation also invites and enforces this new awareness.

Shavasana, or relaxation, is done at the end of every class. Shavasana means "corpse pose," and it involves lying on the floor like a corpse, totally immobile, while methodically releasing every remaining bit of tension in the body.

This can be difficult for some people. It's challenging because we are so used to *doing.* If we are not doing something, then we're sleeping. But shavasana is not sleep. Shavasana is a kind of *undoing.* It's actively letting everything go. It's releasing all of the burdens of the body and mind. It's allowing everything to get very quiet internally without falling into the unconscious state of sleep.

Although it's the least impressive-looking pose, shavasana is considered the most important part of asana practice. This may come as a surprise to some people. And yet it's not hard to fathom the relevance of relaxation. After all, most of us desperately need to relax.

The problem is that we've forgotten how. We're so used to being in constant motion, to responding to the many demands that assault us on a daily basis, that even when we're exhausted we can have trouble stopping. We tend, instead, to resort to sedating ourselves—with food, drugs, alcohol, television, or any number of other things—just to slow down a bit.

This sort of behavior is not very conducive to health. Some people fall into obviously addictive and lethal behaviors, but many people are developing addictions, just by a slower route. Over time, less extreme addictions deplete our systems, too, and contribute to other serious health problems. So, from the standpoint of health alone, learning to relax is key so that we don't have to kill ourselves with self-destructive attempts to relax. Shavasana's real purpose, though, is not just to sustain life, but to put us directly in touch with the mystery of life itself.

How does this happen? When we relax, we start to realize that this body-mind we occupy is not totally under our control. Yes, there are some things we can change; we've experienced this through yoga practice. But as we lie in corpse pose, we realize that something else—something beyond our control—is keeping us alive. Who is it that is keeping our breath going? And who is it that is keeping a steady stream of thoughts running through our minds? We may find ourselves asking these questions and not being able to answer them. What it comes down to is that this body-mind with which we are so identified is not all that we are; within us there is a source of life that animates us.

This realization can be a great relief. It lets us feel less burdened. We feel less responsible for holding it all together. We realize that we can relax into this thing that is greater than ourselves—in fact, that's the only sensible thing to do, because this life source just *is*. We can rest and trust in it.

When we let go in this way, truly allowing ourselves to get quiet, we can directly experience the mystery that gives life to us and everything that exists. This mysterious source is the Self—or whatever you choose to call it. When we get this—that the Self is both in us and in everyone and everything else—and when we sense it at a deeper, more intuitive level, we start to feel very connected with the world. We feel more at one with life itself.

This peaceful feeling gets stronger and more accessible over time. The magic of yoga practice is that after a while, with sustained and consistent effort, this quiet peacefulness takes hold to such a degree that it actually starts seeping into other parts of life. We become aware of feeling differently—of feeling a lot better—as we're working, or driving, or reading, or doing any number of things.

When that happens, it makes it possible to meet the various challenges and obstacles that are a part of day-to-day living with greater equanimity. We're not thrown off-center; it's as if there's a kind of space inside where we can dwell for a moment before we react. We may find that we start to relate to the world differently; our habitual responses to people and situations start to change. So, for example, a person who has needed to rigidly control may (to the relief of family, friends, and colleagues) begin to relax and allow events to unfold more naturally. Or a fearful and shy person might gradually become aware of an underlying sense of power and confidence. Someone's previously scattered, chaotic lifestyle might become focused and directed.

If we go far enough into it, yoga invites change into every aspect of our lives.

Some people feel the effects of yoga quickly and their lives change suddenly. More commonly, though, people make a gradual approach—sometimes in fits and starts—and change slowly.

Change is not always easy and pleasant: as with any enterprise, there are times when difficulties arise. Depending on the condition of the student, the cleansing and healing process that the body undergoes at first can be unpleasant. Someone who smokes, for instance, may start to really feel the negative effects of this habit. Also, as the body starts to change its patterns, old and painful memories are sometimes awakened. This is especially common for people who have been raped or sexually abused, or who have undergone any sort of trauma. In such cases, it's particularly important to have a teacher to help guide the process, pacing it in such a way that it doesn't overwhelm the student, and there is ample time allowed to integrate the changes that are taking place in the body and mind. What's important when these initial challenges arise is to keep the practice continuous and steady so that the positive benefits can keep coming through.

Ultimately, rather than taking us away from the world, yoga can actually make it easier to be *in* the world. It gives practical tools for cultivating and sustaining physical and mental health, and as we feel better, we live our lives better. We become more vital and flowing and more fully engaged in everything we do. At the same time, we're more relaxed about it all.

Yet while our capacities in the external world grow, yoga directs us inward, making us more and more aware of a source inside us—a pool of stillness and quiet that we can trust and reside in. The things of the world become less appealing, because it becomes clear that many of them aren't necessary: they don't have anything to do with this limitless source inside us. In fact, we start to see that the intense stimulation of the senses that we may have once been accustomed to actually takes us away from what's inside us.

Once we make this connection, through trial and error, we keep refining our actions. Of course, we make mistakes: we can't always follow what we know. But yoga practice makes us more steady. It keeps bringing us back to what feels best. It keeps pointing us toward something unchanging, and fundamental, in ourselves. It takes us back to our essential nature.

two

THE ROOTS OF YOGA

Yoga's history is very involved; there are many books to delve into if this aspect interests you. For our purposes, it is useful to understand a bit of yoga's context—to have the sense of where it comes from and how it has evolved.

Yoga began in India, but nobody knows its exact origins or precise age, and much of its earliest history is lost. It definitely predates Christianity and Buddhism, and it is said to be the oldest tradition of self-transcendence. The development of yoga is intimately tied up with India's culture and its most important religious traditions: Hinduism, Jainism, Sikhism, and Buddhism. Interestingly, though yoga is such a highly developed and invaluable part of India's culture, Western scholars have made significant contributions in unraveling the various strands of yoga and understanding the tradition as a whole.

It seems that before the advent of Hatha yoga, which introduced the physical postures and breathing practices, yoga was a system of esoteric knowledge. It was originally an oral tradition, passed down in verse directly from teacher—or *guru*—to disciple. Disciples were required to commit to memory the sacred teachings and rituals and, in this fashion, they were preserved. Given how many hundreds, or even thousands, of verses were contained in many of these teachings, this must have been quite a feat. Though it's less common now, it's still possible to find yogis in India who are capable of recitation of this sort. Fortunately, a number of texts have also been recorded in written form—and translated—and so they're somewhat accessible to the rest of us.

The oldest known collection of sacred knowledge, the *Vedas,* or *Vedic hymns,* go back to somewhere between 4000 and 2000 B.C.E., making yoga at least 4,000 years old. These 1,028 hymns grew out of sacred visions that were articulated by *rishis,* or seers. Through the *Vedas* we're given a sense of the early metaphysical ideas and ritualism of ancient yoga. In *The Yoga Tradition,* Georg Feuerstein quotes Shri Aurobindo, whom he calls one of India's modern seers: "[The *Vedas*] is an inspired knowledge as yet insufficiently equipped with intellectual and philosophical terms. We find a language of poets and illuminates to whom all experience is real, vivid, sensible, even concrete, not yet of thinkers and systematizers to whom the realities of the mind and soul have become abstractions. . . . Here we have the ancient psychological science and the art of spiritual living of which the *Upanishads* are the philosophical outcome."

As Feuerstein explains it, later sections of the *Vedas* came to be considered less appropriate for the common person; they were meant for ascetics who were pursuing their spiritual practices in solitude. They were a precursor to what Feuerstein describes as the even more esoteric *Upanishads,* which ushered yoga into a more ascetic mode.

The *Bhagavadgita* came later and is described by some as the oldest complete yoga work; it's dated from 500 to 400 B.C.E. The *Bhagavadgita* is a long poem that presents yoga through a dialogue between the god Krishna and the warrior prince Arjuna. It is one of the more readable yoga texts.

All of these texts emerged in what is called the "Preclassical" period of yoga. Toward the end of this period, the Buddha was born—his birth is guessed to have been around 563 B.C.E. The Buddhist movement was in part a reaction to the rigidity of contemporary spiritual practices, which had become lifeless and unappealing to many people. Buddhism did take on certain yogic practices, however, and these later developed into Buddhist versions of yoga.

Some time in the fourth century B.C.E., Alexander the Great invaded India and, although his power was short-lived, there seems to have been some overlap—and subsequent mixing—of Greek and Indian cultures. As Rick Fields explains in his history of Buddhism, *How the Swans Came to the Lake,* there were towns that, at Alexander's death, became "centers of a new hybrid Graeco-Buddhist civilization."

After Alexander's death, India recovered its power and diplomatic relations were established between Greece and India. At this time Megasthenes, a Greek ambassador to the Indian court, authored a book on India's history, making India's culture somewhat accessible—even if not entirely comprehensible—to Westerners. Although the book does not contain much information about the spiritual practices of Indians—the problems of language must have been prohibitive—scholars say that there is at least mention of the sages and forest-dwellers who were the early practitioners of yoga.

Over time, ties between Greece and India weakened. It was not until the thirteenth century C.E. that the West made overtures toward India again. In the meantime, from somewhere around the time of Christ's birth up until the seventh century, yoga entered what is called its "Classical" stage. This is defined by the *Yoga Sutras,* a series of short verses compiled by a sage named Patanjali. In the *Yoga Sutras,* the ideas of yoga were systematized in a form that was truly coherent. This text is considered one of the most significant and is by far the most studied yoga text.

Patanjali remains a mysterious figure; nothing definitive is known about him. He probably lived some time in the second century C.E. (although there is some argument around this dating, due to the fact that there were several Patanjalis who lived between 200 B.C.E. and 200 C.E.). Georg Feuerstein points out in *The Yoga Tradition* that it's reasonable to assume that Patanjali was a yoga master and that he probably headed a yoga school of some kind. Feuerstein also writes that many different references are made to the *Yoga Sutras* in scriptures from other philosophical traditions, indicating that Patanjali's school was actually quite influential at one time.

What's known as "Postclassical" yoga, from about the seventh to the seventeenth centuries, brought some big changes to yoga. Tantra yoga emerged at this time, ushering in a new and radical approach that was much more inclusive. Lower-caste people and women were included, and goddess worship was introduced. The whole attitude toward the body—which had previously been seen as despicable and unclean—changed dramatically during this period. It was out of this new physical orientation that Hatha yoga developed.

HOW YOGA CAME WEST

European colonization of India began in the fifteenth century, with the Portuguese, Dutch, French, and English variously controlling centers of trade. Colonists were interested in making use of India for economic gain; there was also considerable effort made to convert Indian people to Christianity, and many terrible atrocities were committed against Indians. India was seen predominantly as a strange and exotic place, with little of substance to offer the West besides its goods. This attitude came to be strongly challenged, though, by an Englishman named Sir William Jones.

In 1783, Jones was appointed to the Supreme Court that was established by the English in India to, among other things, protect the interests of the natives. Jones was a brilliant lawyer who was also renowned for his considerable linguistic talents: he knew Latin, Greek, French, and Spanish and had also studied Arabic, Persian, and Turkish. He had an avid interest in India and had sought a suitable position there—and been thwarted—for years. When he was finally able to go, he launched himself into the work for which he is best known.

His influence was substantial. According to Fields, "Men before him had given accounts, more or less accurate, of what they had seen in the Orient, but it was not until William Jones completed his work in India that the scientific study of Oriental art and philosophy could be said to have even begun."

Jones founded the Royal Asiatic Society, which was dedicated in a very broad way to the study of Asian culture. With some effort, he persuaded someone to teach him Sanskrit and, because of the breadth of his linguistic knowledge, he was able to deduce that European languages and Sanskrit had enough similarities to have actually come from the same source. Jones is also credited for important translations of Sanskrit and Persian works, including the first translations of the Sufi poet Rumi. But, most important, argues Fields, Jones saw "with a historical analogy that has proved prophetic that the translation and study of Asiatic literature could come to play the same role in the modern world that the rediscovery of the Greek and Latin classics did in the renaissance of fifteenth- and sixteenth-century Europe."

The beginnings of this "renaissance" sprang up later in nineteenth-century New England in a movement that came to be known as Transcendentalism. Bronson Alcott, the father of Louisa May Alcott (who authored *Little Women*), was part of this circle. He practiced vegetarianism and ran an alternative school for children. The more familiar Transcendentalists are clergyman Ralph Waldo Emerson, Henry David Thoreau, the author of *On Walden Pond,* and poet Walt Whitman, who wrote *Leaves of Grass.* Anyone who has studied *Leaves of Grass* may recall Whitman's writing style, in which there's a kind of unrelenting inclusiveness of all things. This style essentially expresses that ecstatic state of union that yoga aspires to.

There doesn't seem to have been any organizing principle for the Transcendentalists except a common search for something "new," which they found to some degree in the very ancient philosophies of India. Because there weren't any Indians in the West yet, the Transcendentalists' knowledge of India came strictly through books, many of them authored by Jones. The *Bhagavadgita* had also been translated by this time, and this text was passed around by some within the circle. All of this Eastern influence seems to have nourished a lively and creative American community and set the stage for yoga's emergence in the West.

In September 1893, Chicago hosted the World Parliament of Religions—a huge event, requiring the construction of a whole city. There had never been anything quite like it before and, by the sound of it, it was a spectacular event. It was dominated by Christians, but there were delegates of various Asian countries, too, including Swami Vivekananda from India. Vivekananda, described as one of the more charismatic presenters, was well received. It was through him that Americans were exposed to yoga for the first time.

Following Vivekananda's visit, there was a trickle of other Indians who came and shared their teachings with small but growing numbers of interested seekers. One of the earlier teachers was Paramahansa Yogananda, who founded the Center for Self-Realization in Los Angeles in 1925. He also wrote a popular book called *The Autobiography of a Yogi*. This book is a fascinating story about his relationship with his teacher and his own development as a practitioner and teacher of yoga, both in India and in the United States.

At the time that Yogananda and others were reaching out to Americans on their own soil, a yogi named Krishnamacharya was at work in India. Krishnamacharya is considered by many people to have had the strongest influence on Western yoga. Although he did not come to the West himself, before he died in 1989 at the age of 101, a number of Westerners reached him, including Indra Devi, one of the first Western women to study and teach yoga. Krishnamacharya's influence, though, is said to have been primarily through his training of the teachers who themselves became some of the principle teachers of Westerners.

Born in India in the late nineteenth century, Krishnamacharya came from a long line of yogis and had begun his study of yoga as a young child. He went on to learn many languages and to acquire the equivalent of seven Ph.D.s in subjects as diverse as law, astronomy, and philosophy. He spent seven years studying with a teacher in a Tibetan cave and was capable of stopping his breath and heartbeat for minutes at a time. (This extraordinary feat was documented by a team of European medical experts.) For a number of years, before India's independence, he ran a yoga school that was financed by a maharaj. In his time, Krishnamacharya was very highly respected, and he was much sought after for his medical knowledge and healing powers.

The teachers who studied with Krishnamacharya have educated—and continue to educate—thousands of Americans and students from other countries, who have in turn spread the message of yoga all over the world. These teachers include his brother-in-law, the well-known B. K. S. Iyengar, who has founded some 200 yoga schools around the world. Iyengar has done much to make yoga accessible, and Iyengar yoga is probably the best-known form of yoga in the West. Pattabhi Jois, another student of Krishnamacharya, is responsible for disseminating what's commonly called Ashtanga yoga; this style has also become quite popular, especially in the United States. Krishnamacharya's own son, T. K. V. Desikachar, has trained many American and European teachers in the style of his father. He runs a school that was started while his father was still living, and he's authored a number of very accessible books on yoga and healing.

A NEW YOGA

Yoga in the West has continued to evolve to serve the needs of those practicing it. Historically, men were the main practitioners. Now, however, there are more female than male practitioners—at least in the West. So prenatal yoga, for instance, has been developed as a result of Western women's desire to reclaim the birth experience, as well as their general curiosity about yoga. Postpartum yoga classes, which cater to the special needs of new mothers, have also been developed and have flourished in the West.

Restorative yoga—designed for students needing a very passive practice—is rooted in Iyengar's teaching, but was taken further by an American who called on her yoga training as well as her education in physical therapy and her experience as a working mother. Phoenix Rising Yoga Therapy is a new form that evolved out of Kripalu yoga. And there are also combinations of yoga and other disciplines that go by names like Yoga Movement or Yoga Flow.

This willingness to change and experiment is typically American, and it has led to some very practical and useful innovations.

The hazard of becoming too experimental, though, is that the traditions get lost or so mixed up that nobody knows what's what any longer. Some people are very concerned that yoga is being tampered with too much, and that what is being called "yoga" really isn't yoga at all any more.

Many people argue, though, that some adaptations are necessary. After all, our lives are different here than they were in ancient India. In any case, what will be most important is *your* experience as you investigate the world of yoga. If you find something that works for you, perhaps it does not matter how true to tradition it is. On the other hand, if you want a class that closely follows the spiritual teachings, you'll want to be more discriminating in your search.

three

THE YOGA PATH

Because yoga has been around for a long time, it has had the chance to develop many different styles, each with its own methods. Hatha yoga, which works with the body, is only one branch. There are several others. Several of the main ones are *Jnana* yoga, *Bhakti* yoga, *Karma* yoga, *Mantra* yoga, and *Raja* yoga.

In Jnana yoga—the yoga of wisdom—the seeker approaches self-realization through knowledge. With a teacher's guidance, yoga texts are studied, discussed, and reflected upon. Gradually, the student comes to a deeper understanding of his or her real nature. This approach is said to be one of the most difficult, best suited for people who have strong intellects.

At the other end of the spectrum is Bhakti yoga, which is devotional. Here, a seeker proceeds not through knowledge but through an unconditional surrender of the heart. This is the path of love exemplified by mystics like Kabir and Mirabai. The recently deceased Pakistani singer Nusrat Fateh Ali Khan can also be considered a yogi of the Bhakti tradition.

Karma yoga is the yoga of selfless action. This form involves active participation in the world—not for one's own gain, but to bring about more harmony in the world. Mohandas Gandhi and Mother Teresa are recognized as Karma yogis.

Mantra yoga involves the repetition of a mantra—a sacred sound, or syllable—that is given to the student by the teacher. The mantra is practiced in a particular way, specified by the teacher, and, like the other yogas, eventually leads to self-realization. Most readers will have heard of T. M., or transcendental meditation, which was popular in the '70s and '80s; this practice also involves the repetition of a mantra.

Raja yoga offers still another way. *Raja* means "king," and Raja yoga can be translated as the yoga of the "royal road." In this form, liberation is sought through stilling the fluctuations of the mind; once the mind is able to focus without distraction on a single object, the state of yoga is achieved. Raja yoga, which is also called "Classical yoga," was shaped by the *Yoga Sutras,* which give us some of the most extensive information on yoga practice.

Hatha yoga differs from the other systems in that it deals specifically with the body. Although Hatha yoga is a complete system with its own text, the *Hatha Yoga Pradipika,* it is also seen as a stepping stone, or complement, to Raja yoga. Hatha yoga aims to still the fluctuations of the breath, but this is done in order to quiet the mind—as in Raja yoga. The *Yoga Sutras,* then, make up part of a Hatha yoga student's study.

For yoga to provide a way for its practitioners to live life freely and fully, it must look at the sources of human problems. Why is it that we suffer? The *Yoga Sutras* examine this enormous question and provide some answers—and solutions—in what is considered one of the most systematic and elegant yoga texts available to us. These verses inquire into the nature of mind and give specific strategies for quieting and eventually mastering it.

The *Yoga Sutras* are not long—there are only 195 verses (some editions have 196)—but they are dense and packed with a great deal of theoretical and practical information. Serious students of yoga read the *Sutras* and study them, not once but many times over.

The *Sutras* are organized into four sections: the "chapter on ecstasy," the "chapter on the path," the "chapter on the powers," and the "chapter on liberation."

The text starts with a very clear definition of yoga. One translation reads, "Yoga is the restriction of the fluctuations of consciousness." Another translation is, "Yoga is the ability to direct the mind exclusively toward an object and sustain that direction without any distractions."

That object is not defined: it can be anything, whether physical or not. In other words, the focus could be on something as visible as the flame of a candle. Or it could be on the movement of the breath. The focus could also be directed toward an idea, such as how to solve a mathematical problem or how to understand the growth of plants. The focus can also be God, or the Self.

It is not hard to fathom that this state in which the mind is totally free of distractions is a desirable one. Some people can enter it without much difficulty. But how many of us can stay there for any length of time? The *Sutras* tell us that there are some rare individuals who seem to be born in a fully realized yogic state and that these unusual people don't need to practice. Most of us, however, have to work at stilling and focusing our minds and the *Sutras* give us guidelines for doing this.

If we are going to undertake to still the mind, it is helpful to understand some things about the mind's nature. The mind is a complicated organism, capable of many different sorts of activity. These activities, according to the *Yoga Sutras,* can either be useful to us, moving us toward a more focused state, or they can impede us, sending us into a more scattered state. The mind's activities are broken down into five different classifications: comprehension, misapprehension, imagination, deep sleep, and memory. It is largely through misapprehension—a misinterpretation of what is perceived—that we err. This is called *avidya.*

All of us can probably think of numerous situations in which this has happened. An example is when we wake up frightened in the middle of the night, thinking someone is trying to break in, but it turns out to be just the wind banging a tree branch against the house. Or perhaps we misunderstand what someone tells us and unintentionally start a rumor, passing incorrect information along. Likewise, we may have a hunch about something but don't follow it, only to discover that in fact we were right in the first place. These kinds of things happen all the time.

When we take something to be other than what it actually is, we respond inappropriately. Responding inappropriately can be harmful to us or others, producing suffering, or what's called in Sanskrit *duhkha*. As humans, we continually get stuck in a cycle of avidya and duhkha. How can we avoid avidya in the first place? The first step, the *Sutras* say, is to look at the situation more closely, considering what causes our misunderstanding.

One aspect of avidya has to do with our identity, or the ego. We are constantly referring to ourselves as if this "I" were one solid, unchanging thing. But the fact is that everything about us changes all the time: we have changing moods, changing activities, changing thoughts. Our bodies change all the time, too: one day we have clear skin, the next day a pimple erupts. In fact, it's said that our cells over the course of seven years change completely: cellularly, the body you occupy as you read this page is different from the one you were in seven years ago. So, given all this change, who is this "I"? The *Sutras* tell us that our identification with the ego, or body-mind, is incorrect. The body-mind is not who we really are. Or, more accurately, it's not *all* that we are.

Part of our false understanding can also come from excessive attachment or desire. We've all had the experience of wanting something badly: a new job, a pair of shoes, or a piece of jewelry, for example. Or our desire can be for an activity, like eating a rich meal. When we finally get the thing we were after, we may derive some pleasure from it. That pleasure may even last for a while. But sooner or later, it goes away. Then we find ourselves feeling dissatisfied and wishing for something else. When we fall into this cycle, we make the mistake of believing that an object or an activity that stimulates our senses in some way will fulfill us—but this is not so.

Another aspect of avidya involves a dislike or aversion that is so extreme as to be unreasonable. Racist attitudes stem from avidya. A deep dislike of a certain person can also be the result of avidya. These powerful feelings sometimes overwhelm us because of a past experience that was unpleasant or painful and left a mark in our psyches. Even though the experience is over, we continue to react in the same way.

Still another aspect of avidya is insecurity or fear—especially of the future. The future is frightening to many of us because it is unknown. No matter how confident we may be, we still can't completely anticipate what is ahead for us. Nor do we know how much more time we have on the Earth. Our own death is the greatest unknown, and because we are so identified with the body-mind container we are in, we think that in death we will cease to exist.

This fear is universal and it is said to be one of the most difficult obstacles set in our paths. In fact, most of us experience all of the states of avidya, so there is nothing to be ashamed of. But as long as there is avidya, our actions may be wrong—and they will produce duhkha, or suffering—because they are founded on an incorrect perception of things.

These aspects of avidya—identifying with our ego, excessive attachments, aversion, and insecurity—can be thought of as mental habits. They are the result of our conditioning; we haven't been taught to question these habits, so there's no reason we should think differently. We're simply used to reacting in certain ways, and that's what we continue to do until it occurs to us to try something else.

In order to change a habit, we have to first recognize the habit: we have to see what we're doing. We have to become aware of our automatic responses; only then we can start to see that there might be an alternative. So, in the case of avidya, we have to first be cognizant of the fact that our perception of things is not always accurate. Then we can consider that there might be a different way of perceiving.

The alternative that yoga presents is called the purusha. Purusha, meaning "perceiver" or "seer," is the part of us that is there—perhaps almost obscured by our cloudy perceptions, but there, nonetheless—that can see with total clarity. Unlike the ever-changing mind, from which we think we're getting reliable and correct information, the purusha is constant, unchanging, and totally accurate. We might identify this part of ourselves as soul; Buddhists call it Big Mind.

This is not as abstract as it may sound, because all of us have had experiences of purusha. At one time or another we've heard a voice telling us what to do or had a flash of intuition informing us about something. These are inexplicable moments of just pure knowing. They are instances of purusha. Yoga works to undo avidya—all the habits of faulty understanding that we have—so that the purusha can shine through and we can be directed more and more by this in-dwelling intelligence.

How do we do this? Consider what states of mind might invite experiences of purusha and what states of mind make it impossible. Everyone's had the experience of feeling slow and leaden. Likewise, there's the opposite experience of being hyper and full of too much energy. These states are given names in the *Yoga Sutras:* they are *tamas* and *rajas,* respectively. Both of these states are unbalanced and neither one feels good. The ideal state lies somewhere in the middle: it is called *sattva,* or clarity. When we are in a sattvic state, avidya has less power over us, and the purusha—which is itself beyond the mind—can more easily be recognized and felt.

Experiencing the purusha is a state of grace that we cannot force. However, we can continually work to make the conditions

for it to arise as favorable as possible. The *Sutras* tell us that our
job in life is to cultivate a balanced, sattvic state. Our progress
depends on our practice of asanas and pranayama, on our ongoing inquiry into ourselves, and on the overall quality of our
efforts. The *Sutras* give us a kind of map to follow and anticipate some of the detours we may take and how we may be able
to get ourselves back on track.

THE EIGHT LIMBS OF YOGA

The basic guidelines of the *Sutras* are outlined in a series of
steps, or stages, called "the eight limbs of yoga." There is a pro-
gression through these stages: one stage prepares for the next.
And yet there is no "graduation" from any stage—at least not
until the final state of *samadhi,* self-realization, has been perma-
nently attained. In other words, the eight limbs are guidelines,
or states of mind, which are continuously observed or experienced. Also, they don't exist independently of one another, so
one may be experienced concurrently with another.

The eight limbs start at the most basic level, directing our behavior toward the outside world; then they guide us in our attitudes toward ourselves, becoming more refined with each stage.
They are:

1 *Yama* (discipline)—the guidelines for our actions in the external world;

2 *Niyama* (restraint)—the guidelines governing our actions and attitudes toward ourselves;

3 *Asana* (posture)—the practice of physical postures;

4 *Pranayama* (breath control)—the practice of breath control and exercise;

5 *Pratyahara* (sense withdrawal)—the withdrawal and control of the senses;

6 *Dharana* (concentration)—the focus and concentration of the mind in a direction, toward a particular object;

7 *Dhyana* (meditation)—a meditative state in which there is the ability to interact continuously with the object of focus;

8 *Samadhi* (ecstasy)—the complete, uninterrupted absorption with the object of the mind's focus.

Yama

Yama, the first limb of yoga, is the basic foundation for any practice of yoga. Yama means "discipline" and it directs our attention to our behavior in the world and gives us guidelines for our actions. It consists of moral principles that are universal: *ahimsa* (nonviolence); *satya* (truth telling); *asteya* (non-stealing); *brahmacharya* (continence); and *aparigraha* (non-coveting).

To practice ahimsa means more than to just abstain from violence; it also means to consider all beings and to cultivate an attitude of love and kindness toward others. A person practicing ahimsa understands that all life is precious, and that he or she must help those who aren't as well off. Someone who takes this attitude toward the world is loved and trusted.

Satya, or truth telling, involves refraining from the obvious: obscenity and lies. It can be thought of in Buddhist terms as "right speech," and comprises all forms of communication, whether written, spoken, or physical. The practice of satya means being thoughtful in how we communicate. As we all know, clear communication requires that we be sensitive and alert, and we are well rewarded when we succeed.

Non-stealing—asteya—tells us to resist our desires for things that do not belong to us. Taken a little further, aparigraha, or non-coveting, directs us to resist taking the things we don't really need—to make our lives as simple as possible. When we practice these rules well, we win people's trust and find we are given all the things we need.

Brahmacharya, or continence, is sometimes misunderstood. In the technical sense, brahmacharya means celibacy. For men, it is thought that the loss of semen depletes the body, while retention of semen gives it life: sex, therefore, can be an obstacle. In fact, though, many yogis have married and raised families, and this phase of life is even recommended. The rule of brahmacharya, then, can be interpreted as a more general practice of self-restraint and moderation. With this principle firmly in place in all aspects of living, we experience optimal energy and vitality.

Niyama

The second limb, niyama, offers guidelines for how we relate to ourselves. These principles are *shaucha* (purity or cleanliness); *santosa* (contentment); *tapas* (ardor or austerity); *svadhyaya* (study of the Self); *ishvara pranidhana* (dedication to the Lord).

The first rule of cleanliness, or shaucha, refers to the body, the mind, and the environment. The body is seen as a container for the spirit, and as such it needs to be cared for. It needs to be housed in a clean space and kept clean externally as well as internally: the right food and the right exercise—asana practice combined with pranayama—keep the body's inner workings running smoothly. Krishnamacharya's son, T. K. V. Desikachar, points out that saucha can also be thought of as an ongoing process of discerning between what in ourselves is changing and therefore in need of "maintenance"—in other words, our bodies, emotions, and thoughts—and what is *unchanging*—that essential part of ourselves that needs no cleaning whatsoever: the purusha.

Santosa, contentment, is the practice of accepting what we have, even if it doesn't meet our expectations. It's being happy with what is ours and recognizing that the things we don't have will not in and of themselves make us happy.

The root of tapas means "to blaze" or "to burn." Tapas refers to the process of burning away the impurities in our bodies and minds—the things that we don't need and that stand in our way. This is done through asana and pranayama practices; it is also achieved through watching what we eat.

Svadhyaya—study of the Self—refers to the process of looking at ourselves and inquiring into the relationship we have with ourselves and with the rest of the world. This can mean observing and assessing our own progress. It also involves educating ourselves, and reflecting on ourselves, through the study of sacred literature.

Finally, ishvara pranidhana refers to dedication to the Lord. This definition can be problematic for people who have no connection with a personal God. If that's the case for you, all you need do is recognize that you are not all-powerful and that there is a creative source greater than yourself. This source is what gave you life and brought everything else into existence as well. With this awareness, you can live your life by making your best efforts at whatever you do, while leaving the end results to something else.

Asana

The third limb of yoga is asana practice—the practice of postures and movements designed for certain purposes. Chapter 4 is dedicated to this aspect of yoga, which for Westerners often provides the ground for the experience of yoga. Asana practice helps bring the body into a more healthy and sensitive state and it introduces the most important posture: relaxation. The practice of relaxation puts us into a more meditative frame of mind in preparation for pranayama.

Pranayama

In Hatha yoga, the breath is seen as the vehicle for freedom. In asana practice, some teachers emphasize the breath more than others, but awareness of the breath is an inevitable result of practicing the postures themselves. Breath control begins to be developed at this stage.

In the formal practice of pranayama, instead of focusing on creating certain positions with the body, the mind is directed exclusively toward the breath. This is done by trying to control the breath through specific breathing exercises, which are done in a comfortable seated position. With pranayama, the mind becomes more and more focused; it becomes immersed in the breath. These breathing exercises lead naturally into the next stages: pratyahara, dharana, dhyana, and samadhi.

Pratyahara, Dharana, Dhyana, Samadhi

Pratyahara is the withdrawal of the senses. It's also defined as the control or restraint of the senses. This stage ushers in a new relationship to the senses, in which they simply, over time, lose their power over our actions. In this stage, we're no longer driven or distracted by our desires. Pratyahara is the natural outcome of the physical practices—asanas and pranayama—in which the mind's attention keeps being directed inward. But it is also the result of consciously observing the rules of yama and niyama, in which we try to curb our desires for things we don't really need: we try to bring moderation and balance to all our actions.

Dharana takes the process a little further. Dharana is the stage in which the senses are no longer obstacles and the mind is free to start making contact with the object on which it's trying to focus. It's at this stage that we begin to become more "one-pointed." Many people begin to experience this during pranayama practice. Of course, since the object can be anything, you have no doubt experienced this state yourself when you initiate an activity that you've wanted to do for awhile. Say, for example, that you finally stop snacking or puttering around the house and begin to focus on doing your taxes. That's an example of dharana.

Dhyana occurs when the mind's focus is undisturbed, and there is a *continual* connection with the object. The activities of the mind are concentrated solely on the object. Again, some people experience this state during pranayama. To go back to the last example, this state might be characterized by being able to sit and work for three hours on your taxes.

Finally, samadhi occurs when the mental involvement is so complete that there is no longer any awareness of the self: we lose our sense of identity, becoming completely merged with the object of our attention. Even this state can be broken down and classified in different ways. There is the category of "conscious ecstasy," describing different possible ecstatic states in which there is a *partial* transcendence of the Self. Some people go in and out of this state during very deep meditation. Then there is "supraconscious ecstasy," which is impossible for ordinary people to imagine, because it goes totally beyond any sort of everyday experience. What we do know is that it's a state so blissful as to be beyond any description. It's also a state that very few people attain, and it's said that those who do achieve it are often not very visible; these people are not particularly interested in drawing attention to themselves.

The eight limbs of yoga give guidelines for progressively refining our attention so that we can reach some state of samadhi. Of course, as with any endeavor, there is rarely a straight path toward the goal. One of the potential stumbling blocks has to do with the powers attained in advanced yoga practice.

THE *SIDDHIS,* OR SPECIAL POWERS

Many people are unaware of the superhuman powers, or *siddhis,* that some yogis attain once they've achieved a certain level of mastery over the mind. One of the chapters in the *Yoga Sutras* is devoted to this subject. At this stage, anything that these yogis direct their minds toward can be deeply known. Thus,

"[Through the practice of constraint] upon the strengths, [he acquires] the strength of an elephant and so on" (3.24). In other yogic literature there are accounts of yogis who can read minds, heal the deathly ill, manifest themselves in more than one place at a time, live without food or drink, stop their own heartbeat, and perform many other miraculous feats.

In *Return of the Rishi*, Deepak Chopra describes witnessing one such event during his medical school training. Many miraculous feats are also recounted in Yogananda Paramahansa's popular book, *Autobiography of a Yogi*. Yogananda himself possessed some of these powers. In a note at the end of his book are some extracts from a notarized mortuary report regarding Yogananda's condition after his death on March 7, 1952. "The absence of any visual signs of decay in the dead body . . . offers the most extraordinary case in our experience. . . . No physical deterioration was visible in his body even twenty days after death. No indication of mold was visible on his skin, and no visible desiccation (drying up) took place in the body tissues. This state of perfect preservation of a body is, so far as we know from mortuary annals, an unparalleled one."

It's been suggested that these extraordinary powers are displayed from time to time mostly in order to inspire faith in the unbelieving. These powers are definitely not to be mistaken for the end goal. They are just tricks—distractions, in fact—and for that reason, many yoga masters refuse to teach them to others.

The danger, of course, is that these superhuman powers can be very seductive; some practitioners get attached to them and then never proceed to the real goal, which is self-realization.

For most of us, however, the difficulties and obstacles that arise are more mundane. The *Sutras* anticipate these and give some suggestions for how they might be overcome.

OBSTACLES IN OUR PATHS

The obstacles we are most likely to encounter in yoga practice are, according to Desikachar's translations in *The Heart of Yoga,* illness, lethargy, doubt, haste or impatience, resignation or fatigue, distraction, ignorance or arrogance, lack of concentration, inability to take a new step, and loss of confidence. He explains that these usually show up in symptoms like self-pity, negative thinking, physical difficulties, or breathing problems.

Fortunately, there are many steps we can take to help ourselves. First of all, when we find ourselves having difficulty, this is an opportunity to seek out the guidance of our teacher. The word *guru,* after all, translates as someone who sheds light where there is darkness. A teacher may have some insights or perspective on our situation that we can't figure out by ourselves.

The *Sutras* also advise us to be friendly, positive, and compassionate toward other people. Extending ourselves in this way may draw us out of any self-pity or negativity we're stuck in. Practicing pranayama correctly can help counteract the breathing problems we may be experiencing. And looking deeply into how our senses impact us can also be helpful.

Desikachar elaborates on this last suggestion. He says it may be illuminating to ask ourselves questions like, "How do I observe things?" or "How do I hear sounds?" What is important is not so much what answers come to us, but that we simply take the step to quiet and redirect the mind by asking ourselves these questions.

It may also be instructive to talk to someone who's gone through what we're going through: it's quite possible that our experience is not unique and that someone else may have experience that is very relevant to us.

We can also turn to our dreams to inform us: sometimes making an effort to remember our dreams and considering their possible meanings will yield answers.

Sometimes, though, we can know what might be good for us and still not be able to do it. If this is the case, it may be best just to resort to something that has worked for you in the past when you've felt blocked, or uninspired, or stuck in some way. If there are activities you like that you know are soothing—like playing the piano, walking, or reading—try one of those.

In the end, what may get us through is our faith—our basic belief that we will somehow get through our difficulties and succeed in reaching our goals. In the *Sutras,* it is said that "[the supraconscious ecstasy] is close for [those yogins who are] extremely intense [in their practice of Yoga]" (1.21). Further on, it states "Or [supraconscious ecstasy is gained] through devotion to the Lord" (1.23). So it's either through our intense practice or our intense faith in something higher that we succeed. What's important to know is that yoga gives guidelines only. It gives us a technology, but that is only a means. In the end, we each have to make our own way.

four

PRINCIPLES OF YOGA PRACTICE

Your interest in yoga may stem from a desire to heal yourself in some way. Perhaps you have developed problems with your back, neck, or shoulders. Maybe you're finding yourself inordinately stressed out. Or maybe you're in pretty good health but you're curious about what could make you feel even better.

Whatever your state, you're probably at least somewhat aware of the effects of gravity and time on your body. Most of us don't have the same capacities that we had as kids. Unless we're exercising regularly and in a balanced way, our bodies lose their strength and tighten up with age. When these trends continue without being addressed, we gradually become less happy in our bodies and we tend to neglect ourselves more. It can be a slow process; often we don't pay attention until an obvious problem presents itself.

Regular yoga practice keeps us strong and limber and boosts our immune systems, so that we're much less vulnerable to injury or illness. And if we're not in a healthy, vital state when we begin, yoga can eventually get us there. Yoga gives us a way to examine where we are and slowly change ourselves for the better.

Given the right attention, many health problems clear up. And many people, once they make yoga practice a regular part of their lives, find that they feel better than ever.

HOW ASANAS WORK

The asanas make up the physical part of yoga practice. Although you can learn some things from a book, a teacher is essential when you're trying to learn asanas. To benefit fully from a pose, you have to have an understanding of its purpose. Then you have to know how to sufficiently prepare yourself for the pose and how to execute it properly. Some postures, if practiced incorrectly, can lead to injury. A teacher can help you with all of this. What's provided here are some basic principles to give you a general idea of what asana practice is about.

Asanas work by strengthening and toning the body while simultaneously increasing its flexibility and mobility. Usually, people tend to be more developed in one way or the other. Some of us possess a certain amount of strength but we're not very flexible. Others are flexible but have no muscle tone. If you've got some flexibility already, yoga will help you balance that by increasing your strength. And as you become stronger you'll start feeling less weighed down. Your movements in the world will feel more sure, because your body will be more solid. Likewise, if you have strength but no flexibility, yoga will slowly ease the tightness out of your body, and you'll start to feel more free in your movements. So asana practice helps balance strength with flexibility.

Asana practice also works to correct other imbalances in the body. For instance, if you're stronger in one leg than the other, yoga will help your weaker leg "catch up" to the stronger one. Or if one shoulder is more open than the other, yoga will gradually restore range of motion to the tight side. All of us have these imbalances. Yoga makes us more aware of them so that we can take corrective measures—not in the interest of being perfect, but so that we'll feel better.

DIFFERENT KINDS OF ASANAS

Some asanas are done standing in an upright position; some are done seated; and some are done lying on the floor on the stomach, side, or back. Asanas tend either to strengthen some part of the body or to encourage more flexibility in an area. However, many asanas do both: they strengthen one part of the body while simultaneously opening up another. In fact, there are a number of actions going on in the body with each posture, and as you gain experience you'll become more aware of these.

The standing postures usually provide the basics of a yoga practice, and once a beginner understands the proper placement of the feet, legs, and hips for these postures, there are many different standing poses that can be learned. These poses tend to strengthen and energize the body.

Balance poses can also be strengthening and energizing, as they demand that muscles work in a way they may not be accustomed to. A balance pose can be something like standing on one leg, while extending the arms and the free leg in a particular way. Balance poses can be somewhat daunting—especially at first—because they can be quite challenging. What is striking, however, is that with just a little practice, they become much more doable.

There are also asanas called "inverted poses," in which the head is below the heart. These include poses like headstand, shoulder stand, and handstand. These postures are good for circulation because they reverse the normal flow of blood, encouraging its movement into parts of the body that don't normally receive as much blood flow. Inverted postures can also be good for the spine because they reverse the spine's normal relationship to gravity. Some inverted postures are very strengthening to the upper body: the arms, neck, and back. Many of these postures are introduced later in a person's study of yoga, after a certain amount of strength, endurance, and flexibility have already been built up. A number of the inverted poses—like the shoulder stand, for example—need to be approached with caution, as they can be harmful if practiced incorrectly.

Many postures are done on the floor and they can have various effects. Twisting postures increase the mobility of the spine, making it more flexible; they often help to open up the chest as well and aid with digestion. Other floor poses can work to lengthen the spine—as in a seated forward bend. This same posture also stretches and opens the backs of the legs. There are many floor postures that tone the abdominal area, at the same time giving more support to the lower back.

Once there is some familiarity with the poses themselves, then there are many variations that can be explored. Take, for instance, *uttanasana,* which starts in a standing position and involves folding the upper body down toward the legs. Traditionally, this position is done with both legs straight. But as a way to vary the pose, one knee can be bent, while the other remains straight. After this variation is held for a few breaths, the leg positions are switched. Working with variations in this way allows you to investigate different aspects of the poses and can keep your practice from getting mechanical and stale.

SEQUENCING THE POSTURES

As you will see once you start taking yoga classes, there are endless combinations of postures. How postures are sequenced depends on a number of things.

First of all, there's a sensible timing and rhythm in a well-planned yoga practice. The overall structure of a practice session is such that it starts with less strenuous postures and gradually builds up to the more challenging ones. Sufficient time is given for winding down a practice in preparation for shavasana, or relaxation.

There should also be a logic to the sequencing, so that one posture prepares the body in some way for the next. So, for instance, if you're trying to get into a demanding twist, it makes sense to try some milder twists first. Or a series of back-opening postures may be the right way to approach going into a full back bend. This notion of progressing from one pose to another in an orderly way is called *vinyasa.*

Another consideration is this: A pose that takes you deeply in one direction needs to be balanced by a pose that moves you the other way. So, for example, if you twist toward one side of the body, you always want to counter that action by twisting the other way, too. Or if you bend the spine backward, as you would in a back bend, there needs to be movement the other way, going into a pose like a forward bend. The idea is to balance poses with appropriate counterposes.

When you first start taking yoga classes, your mind may not completely follow the reasoning for a class structure. It's not critical that you understand in the beginning; it will become clear in time as you grow more familiar with typical sequencing, and as you become more sensitive to your body and its responses. What's most important is that you keep drawing your attention to what you're doing from moment to moment.

This, in fact, is a very important point. Paying attention is a necessity. For one thing, if you're not, you simply won't be able to do certain things. Balance poses, for example, are completely impossible when the mind is wandering. You're also more likely to injure yourself if you're not attentive.

Suppose you are working with a pose like uttanasana, the standing forward bend mentioned above. As you come into the pose, you notice the smell of bread baking and your mind starts thinking about what you're going to eat when you're done with class. Meanwhile, you've failed to notice that your back is hurting. Because you weren't paying attention, you didn't notice at what point your back started to complain, so you went more deeply into the pose than was really appropriate. Maybe there's only a little bit of strain—or maybe there's a more serious injury—but the point is that we can avoid these things if we're alert.

Bear in mind that what we're doing here is not just mechanically exercising the body so that we can go on to the next thing. We're trying to make ourselves whole through this process: we're trying to bring together the mind, body, and spirit. This is meant to be an enjoyable activity. It may be challenging and hard at times, but it should feel good and you should like doing it. So, during practice, if you catch your mind wandering you can ask yourself why. Are you tired? Bored? Hungry? Fearful? Are you in pain? You can learn something about yourself. Working with your body in this way is just another way of inquiring into yourself and getting information about yourself. In this way, you become increasingly aware of your mental habits and changing states of mind.

THE BREATH

In asana practice, it is not just a matter of getting into a position and then holding your body there; how you breathe is equally important. The breath should be even and deep, without being forced. As you practice you'll start to notice the role of the breath, and you'll see that fluctuations in the breath can affect your concentration. Likewise, changes in your concentration are reflected in the breath. Also, the quality of your breath can give you clues about your state of mind and the way you're going about your practice. For instance, if you notice that your breath is gasping and uneven, that's a clear sign that there is too much effort being put into what you're doing. Similarly, if your breath is barely perceptible, then maybe you need to be doing a posture that will challenge you a little more.

In yoga practice, the breath is generally coordinated in a particular—and natural—way with our movements, so that there's an obvious connection between the two. For example, if you're preparing to go into uttanasana from a standing position, you sweep the arms up overhead as your breath comes in. Then, as you exhale, you fold forward. After you hold yourself there for a number of breaths, you lift yourself back to an upright position as you breathe in. This connection between breath and movement becomes completely second nature after awhile.

There are other ways of working with the breath, too, which may feel less natural in the beginning. One is to start timing your breaths to see if your inhale matches your exhale. Many of us give more time to our inhalations and rush a little during our exhalations. As we practice, we observe this and then try to balance things out, so that the exhalation is just as long as the inhalation.

Another way to work with the breath is to purposefully lengthen the exhalation so that it's significantly longer than the inhalation. We can also retain the breath for a few seconds in between the inhalation and the exhalation. Or another option is to hold the breath out of the body for a few seconds before breathing in again. In fact, there are many different ways of engaging the breath, and over time we get more skilled in working with these variations.

A specific breathing technique that is especially helpful is called the *ujjayi* breath. With the ujjayi breath, the throat is slightly constricted, so that the breath makes an audible sound

57

PRINCIPLES OF

YOGA PRACTICE

as it moves in and out. It sounds a bit like wind going through a tunnel, or the ocean as it moves back and forth along the shore. This breath is particularly useful because of the auditory component: the fact that we can hear ourselves can make it a little easier to notice our breath. So, again, if the breath sounds choppy, we're going beyond our proper limit. If we can't hear ourselves at all anymore, then maybe the mind has wandered.

All of these techniques improve our breathing, and they add another dimension to the postures by intensifying their effects. The breath is an invaluable tool for keeping the attention fixed in the moment. This makes our practice safer and helps us understand that a posture is not just one discrete moment in time: it is a collection of moments in which many things are going on in the body—and the mind—simultaneously. Working with the breath in these various ways makes us more sensitive to the interplay between the mind, the breath, and the body. And once we've become aware in this way, we're more prepared for the later practices of pranayama.

EFFORT AND EASE

A very important consideration in yoga practice is how to balance effort with ease. The *Yoga Sutras* tell us that a posture should be both energetic *and* relaxed. As we've seen, the breath is a good barometer: if you're gasping for breath, or if the breath is ragged and uneven, that's an indication that you are bringing too much effort into your practice. If you are in great pain in a posture, you are definitely trying too hard. If your limbs shake a lot when you're holding a posture, you're probably pushing too much. Too much effort can be counterproductive, leading to stress and strain and possible injury. If you find yourself trying too hard, then it's time to ease up on the posture and see if you can relax into it more instead of trying so hard.

This can be challenging, especially for people who naturally drive themselves and who are used to controlling things. This is a habit of the mind; it's a familiar way of being in the world, and so it's comfortable. See what happens if you catch yourself doing that—and stop. What you'll find—ultimately—is that the goal you are so desperately striving toward actually gets closer when you relax. If you take the time to ease into a posture very slowly, letting it evolve instead of forcing it to, you'll eventually drop more deeply into it. This is a paradox that you can only understand by experiencing it yourself.

At the other end of the spectrum are people who tend to be a little too dull and disengaged as they practice, not bringing enough energy to their actions. This is sometimes true of depressed people. It can also be a habit of people who, for whatever reason, are afraid of trying a little harder. If, as you're practicing a posture, you don't feel much of anything going on, you could probably increase your efforts. Even if you have a natural aptitude for these positions and they feel relatively easy to you, there are always improvements and refinements that can be made. Observe your breath, and if it's very shallow, you're not engaging it enough. Deepen it and see what happens. This alone can flood the body and mind with oxygen, bringing more energy to your whole system.

Like the person who habitually tries too hard, the more disengaged person can find it difficult to change his or her habits. An uninvolved way of being can also be a way of attempting to control—but by containing energy, instead of letting it out. Sometimes as we start to allow more energy to come through us, it can be frightening. It can stir up uncomfortable emotions. Or it can just be alarming, as we realize that maybe there are other possibilities for being in the world.

Most of us vacillate between these two states, at times energetic, at other times dull. It's intelligent to recognize that there are times when we feel less energetic for good reason: maybe we haven't slept enough, or we've been working too hard, or we're recovering from a cold. In such a case, it's entirely appropriate to modify our practice so that we're not overdoing it. A good teacher helps us recognize the state we're in and guides us toward a more balanced way of practicing. And over time it gets easier to recognize for ourselves our inner state, and we become more able to regulate our own practice.

When we start taking yoga classes, it's natural to look around and watch other people to see how they're doing things. Observing other people can be helpful, because we can learn from more experienced practitioners. We can even be inspired by them, too. But we must avoid comparisons of a competitive nature. This is sometimes difficult. In this day and age, we are very competitive and goal-oriented. But yoga is really not at all about looking good. It's not meant to be a performance in any way. This practice is about you. It's a moving meditation with yourself.

MAKING PROGRESS

All of us like to feel that we're progressing. When we progress forward in an obvious way, we feel good; we feel a sense of accomplishment. The problem is that we get attached to that sense of having achieved something, and so when something isn't possible, we feel badly. It can be very devastating for some of us to realize that we just can't do a pose yet: we're not ready. What can be even more maddening is that sometimes a pose that we could do last week is out of reach this week. Not only have we not progressed, we've actually slipped backward!

Yoga teaches us to simply pay attention and work with what we have right now—as opposed to yesterday or tomorrow. We have to be patient, and this requires a certain internal discipline. (Remember that the word *yoga* also translates as "discipline.") The real measure of our progress is how present we can be to ourselves and how skillful we are in testing and negotiating our limits.

Of course, there often *is* a sense of progress, because with practice, we inevitably improve. Postures become more accessible and can be held for longer periods of time. The body is amazingly responsive to even a little bit of attention. When we improve, it's of course easier to want to practice. When we feel we're slipping back, a good teacher can help inspire renewed efforts and can also give us some perspective on how far we really have come.

RELAXATION

Relaxation, or shavasana, follows yoga practice. Some beginning students are tempted to skip this part, especially if relaxation doesn't come easily. But it's important to make the attempt. Physiologically, this is when your body can rest and absorb all that you have been doing with it. More so, relaxation is when you start to really enter the heart of yoga.

If you can do this without falling asleep, so much the better.

In the beginning, though, you *may* fall asleep—and that's OK. It's natural, because so many of us equate relaxation with sleep. We have to learn how to rest without falling asleep, and that can take some time. There are suggestions for how to practice this posture in chapter 7.

PRANAYAMA: BREATH CONTROL

Pranayama, or breath control, is extremely important in many forms of yoga. It is central to Hatha yoga, in which the aim is to still the fluctuations of the breath. Asana practice, which begins to work with the breath, prepares you for this next step, which is more concentrated breath work.

Consider your breath for a moment. You have been breathing since the day you were born. Nobody had to teach you: you just knew how to do it. After many years of breathing, your body still performs this function automatically, without being told. It's a wondrous thing, like the heartbeat. But it's also something over which we do have some control—more so than we may think.

All of us have had the experience of the breath becoming more rapid and shallow when we're frightened. To a degree, we may already know how to calm ourselves by deepening the breath. Once you have been doing asana practice for some time, you will be still more conscious of your breath. You will have some skill in observing it, and you'll be more appreciative of the subtle shifts in your breath and how these affect, and are affected by, your state of mind.

Prana is our life-force, our vitality. Without prana, there is no life; the more prana we have, the more alive we are. With pranayama, we are trying to increase our vitality. We do this by working with the breath to eliminate the impurities in the body. We are also trying to eliminate the impurities—or the excess baggage—in our minds. So we build our prana, our life-force, by using our breath to influence our minds. Pranayama is just another way to get us into a more meditative state.

In the *Hatha Yoga Pradipika,* it is recommended that pranayama practice take place four times a day: in the early morning, at noon, in the evening, and at midnight. This is, of course, completely impractical for most people, so what Iyengar recommends in his book *Light on Yoga* is to practice at least fifteen minutes a day. Pranayama should happen after asana practice, with a short break in between. Like asana practice, you should learn pranayama first from a teacher so that you know how to do the exercises properly.

YOGA AND FOOD

As you immerse yourself more in the practices, you'll find more parts of your life being influenced in one way or another. In particular, you may find yourself more conscious—and curious—about food.

As with any form of exercise, you don't want to eat a big meal just before your yoga practice; this is very hard on the body and impedes the digestive process. It's generally recommended that you practice on an empty stomach, which means timing your practice for three, or perhaps four, hours after eating. If you have a high metabolism or low blood sugar, it may be appropriate to have a light snack an hour or so before practice. As you practice yoga more, the dietary rhythms of your body will become more obvious, and you'll know how to time yourself.

In the West, there is a tendency to overeat and to eat too quickly. Overeating makes the whole system sluggish and inert and can ultimately damage your health if it's habitual. And eating on the run can also tax the digestive system and make it difficult to absorb and assimilate the food's nutrients. It is useful to observe how we approach eating, and to begin to notice how our dietary habits impact our physical and mental states.

Westerners also tend to consume more meat and dairy products than are nutritionally necessary. And, unfortunately, unless these products are organic, they contain high amounts of hormones that can then accumulate in the body and contribute to serious health problems later on.

For these reasons and others, many people who practice yoga become vegetarians, or lacto-vegetarians (who include some dairy products in their diet). There is no need to feel that you should instantly and radically change how you eat, unless, for example, you have a medical emergency and your doctor insists that you immediately cut your fat intake. It's generally most useful to approach dietary changes slowly, and to let the process of change evolve in its own time: you may come to yoga with an unhealthful diet and poor eating habits, and as your body becomes more sensitive, and as its metabolism increases with yoga practice, these habits naturally begin to shift with no special effort on your part. You may begin to notice, perhaps for the first time, that a particular food is making you feel badly, so you stop eating it or you cut down on your intake. Your body may simultaneously start to crave foods with more nutritional substance. Follow these signals and keep observing your food habits; this is all part of the yogic path.

AYURVEDIC PRINCIPLES

The fact that food and the way it is eaten can have a strong impact on the body and the mind has long been recognized in the Indian healing system of *Ayurveda*. Like yoga, Ayurveda has its roots in the Vedic tradition. It is an allopathic medical system that emphasizes prevention of disease by cultivating and maintaining good health through proper diet.

In Ayurveda, foods are understood in terms of the three *gunas*—the three qualities that also exist in our minds: tamas (heaviness), rajas (agitation), and sattva (clarity). So foods that are rich and tamasic—like meat, cheese, and butter—will probably make you feel tired and heavy. It may be appropriate to eat tamasic foods when you feel that you have too much energy and you want to calm yourself down. On the other hand, foods that are rajasic—spicy and fiery-—will perk you up and give you energy when you're feeling low.

Part of yoga practice, then, involves becoming more aware of the effects that different foods have on us. As we start noticing these effects more, we can make more educated choices about how to nourish ourselves. Through diet, we have another tool for clearing our minds.

It is impossible to come up with any set rules around food, except that a healthful, balanced diet is recommended. We each have individual dietary needs, and they can vary from day to day or moment to moment. Sometimes we are good at attending to and following the body's signals; sometimes we fall into old habits. It takes time to change, and if you find yourself indulging in a food that you know is not beneficial, don't berate yourself. It's better to enjoy yourself than poison yourself with derision. The important thing is to keep paying attention, to attune yourself more and more to the subtle shifts in your body and mind, and to respond as best you can.

The *way* that we eat food is just as important as what we eat. For some of us, it is very difficult to clear space in each day to eat slowly and really enjoy our meals; the structure of our lives just doesn't allow it. But as much as possible, we can cultivate more awareness around our food, taking a little more care in how we shop and how we prepare our foods. We can at least sit down when we eat, and once in a while, we can make time in our schedule for a leisurely, relaxed meal.

If you have questions about your diet, you may want to consult with a doctor, nutritionist, or Ayurvedic doctor. Also, if you have an eating disorder, it's wise to seek help from other resources; a therapist or an organization like Overeaters Anonymous can be very helpful.

A few general guidelines:

- Start paying more attention to the ingredients listed on packaging. Many processed foods have additives and preservatives, both of which are toxic to the body. Many of these processed or packaged foods also contain high quantities of salt and sugar.

- Observe how much sugar you eat, including the amount that you consume through packaged and processed foods.

- Notice your intake of salt. If you eat a lot of processed foods or if you eat out a lot, you are probably consuming more salt than you realize.

- Notice how much fat, animal fat in particular, you are consuming. Again, if you often eat out, the chances are high that you are also consuming additives and preservatives. If you are going to eat meat, consider buying organic meat.

- Increase your intake of fruits, vegetables, and whole grains.

- Buy organic fruits, vegetables, and grains if they are available.

- Drink filtered water; there are many damaging chemicals in regular tap water. Drink water between meals.

- Prepare your meals so that they're appealing.

- Avoid eating while standing, reading, or doing some other activity. Make some time for leisurely eating; enjoy your meals.

The practice of yoga invites more attention to everything we do with our bodies. Of course, all of this takes more effort. And as with our yoga practice, we have to balance effort with ease in our day-to-day living. Eat sensibly. Cut yourself slack when you need to. And keep noticing how you feel.

five

FINDING A YOGA CLASS

If your interest is sparked and you think you want to try taking a yoga class, it will be useful to have some idea as to
what's out there and what might work best for you. The kind of
class you'll want depends on your age, your state of health, and
your personality.

As yoga has become more and more popular, it's easier to find
all kinds of classes. Of course, you can begin your search by looking for a studio devoted exclusively to yoga. But you can also find
yoga classes in dance studios, gyms, health clubs, hospitals, and
senior centers. One thing to be aware of is that yoga studios are
set up especially for yoga practice, and so they tend to be cleaner
and better equipped. This is not to say, though, that you can't
find a perfectly good class elsewhere. What's most important is to
find the right yoga style for you and a teacher whom you like—
and there's no telling where good teachers may crop up.

Some yoga studios specialize in one style of yoga. You're just
as likely, though, to find a mixture of classes at any given studio. The kinds of yoga classes that you'll most likely see offered
in studios and health clubs in the United States go by the names

of Hatha yoga, Iyengar yoga, restorative yoga, Ashtanga yoga, prenatal and postpartum yoga, and Kundalini yoga. (Remember that the term *Hatha* is sometimes used generically to denote the practice of physical postures.) You may also run across Bikram, Kripalu, and Tantra yogas. There are others, of course, and sometimes teachers come up with their own names, too, like Yoga Flow or Yoga Movement. Such labels usually indicate a blending of styles, or a mixture of yoga with some other form like dance. Sometimes classes are simply labeled "Beginning," "Intermediate," or "Advanced," and if you come across a class like that, you may have to contact the teacher directly to find out what style the teaching is based on.

The descriptions below should give you some sense of your choices. Be aware, though, that you can't really know what a class is like until you attend it. Even when two teachers use the same names to describe their classes, the classes can actually be quite different. So what may work best is to get a general idea of what style would be likely to suit you, and then start looking around for a teacher.

Iyengar Yoga

Iyengar yoga is probably one of the best-known styles. It gets its name from B. K. S. Iyengar, who has been extremely influential in the yoga movement worldwide. Many of the more established yoga schools in the United States have been founded by people who have studied directly with him. Iyengar is now in his eighties and no longer teaches public classes.

One of Iyengar's achievements has been to use his own body as a kind of laboratory. He's dedicated his life to considering and figuring out for himself what needs to occur in the body to be able to reach certain positions or to move in particular ways. He has thoroughly examined the minutiae of postures and broken them down for others, so that they can know what steps are necessary in order to progress toward the final form of each posture. Iyengar has authored a number of books, one of which, *Light on Yoga,* gives detailed descriptions of the postures. A glance through the magnificent pictures of him in various postures will give you some sense of the physical achievements that are possible with steady yoga practice.

Iyengar is known in particular for his very practical and clever use of props to assist students in their poses. He noticed that some students, in their eagerness to do postures correctly, strained or injured themselves. But these injuries could be avoided by approaching the postures more gradually and safely, with the assistance of a small block, or a strap, or some other prop. With time and practice, a student could work sensibly toward the complete posture, perhaps some day without any external assistance at all.

So a studio that offers Iyengar yoga classes usually has many props to choose from. These include wooden blocks, straps, chairs, bolsters, and blankets; there may also be ropes hanging from walls, or a swing dangling from the ceiling. Should you ever explore Iyengar yoga, you will be astonished at the great variety of uses for something as simple as a wooden block. It can be very exciting and satisfying to make proper use of these tools, because with them poses that were previously impossible become possible.

Iyengar classes often focus on a certain theme. One class might be devoted to poses that open up the hips, while another class might focus more on poses for widening the chest. In Iyengar yoga you begin to understand more consciously how the poses impact the body or how you can work the poses to effect certain changes.

The complaint that people sometimes have about this form is that the use of props can detract from the meditative quality of a class. Imagine having to get up to get a chair, set yourself up in a particular way, then stay in the pose for a certain amount of time, then extract yourself from the position, get up again, put the chair away, and try something different—possibly with yet another prop. Even though there may be a very obvious and useful order to these procedures, they can take away from the flow of a class.

Nonetheless, because of its precision, attention to detail, and slow pace, Iyengar yoga is a terrific form for beginners. This style of yoga does not stop with the body: advanced students go on to delve deeply into other aspects of yoga practice.

Ashtanga Yoga

What's known as "Ashtanga yoga" is also sometimes called Ashtanga Vinyasa, or "Power Yoga." The story goes that the basis of this system was found in a manuscript written on a bundle of palm leaves. The manuscript—which is believed to be between 500 and 1,000 years old—was discovered in a library by Krishnamacharya and one of his students, Pattabhi Jois. Together, they translated it and reassembled the series of postures. Pattabhi Jois became the main proponent of this system and continues to teach it in India. This particular style has become fairly popular in the United States in the past few years.

Ashtanga yoga works with a set series of postures. So, if you take a class in Atlanta, Georgia, you should get the exact same sequencing as you would in Berkeley, California. In the first part of a class, the postures are strung together in one continuous flowing movement—vinyasa—in which the movements are linked with the breath. Throughout the class, the ujjayi breath is practiced: this is the technique of slightly closing the back of the throat as you breathe so that there's an audible, hissing sound. Also, certain *bandhas* are employed: these are techniques for sealing off the body's energy at places where it might "leak." For example, *mula bandha* is the technique of contracting the perineum; instead of flowing outward, the body's energy is channeled up through the spine.

After your body warms up during the first sequences, other sets of postures are introduced, and this time each pose is held for a period of time. The body tends to cool down a little during this stage, so vinyasas are sometimes thrown in to rekindle the body's heat.

One thing that distinguishes Ashtanga from other systems is that it is practiced in a very warm room. Typically, the windows are closed tight and the heat is cranked up high. This creates external heat in addition to the internal heat being generated in the body. Consequently, you sweat—a lot. It's not unusual to finish up a class completely drenched.

This style of yoga is generally appealing to a younger crowd. It can require a lot of energy to do it, and it works best for people who already enjoy a certain basic level of health. It's not appropriate for people who have serious injuries or who are ill.

When you first start out, Ashtanga yoga can be a little intimidating, because everyone else may seem to already know the sequence of moves, and the pace can seem pretty fast. However, the sequences are fairly simple, and it doesn't take long to learn them.

One of the concerns expressed about this type of yoga, though, is that because it moves so quickly—especially in the beginning part of a class—the correct positioning of the body sometimes gets brushed over, and new students don't always learn the basics as thoroughly as they might in a more slowly paced class. As a result, students can get into some bad habits that don't always get corrected and can then lead to injury. This depends a lot on the teacher. If you happen on an introductory Ashtanga course, you'll definitely want to check this out first, as it may break things down a little more slowly and methodically.

Ashtanga certainly has many enthusiastic followers, for a number of reasons. The fact that it's essentially the same routine practiced over and over again (until you're ready to advance to the next level) makes it possible to get into a flow: the sequence of poses becomes automatic, so you can start to focus on refining the movements themselves. Also, once you get into practicing by yourself, you really don't have to make any creative choices about sequencing: you just do what you always do. So Ashtanga yoga appeals to people who like routine and who also appreciate a strong physical challenge, and, if it's practiced in a safe way, there will be significant positive changes in strength, flexibility, and energy in a short period of time.

Kundalini Yoga

Kundalini yoga was introduced to this country in the 1960s by an Indian Sikh calling himself Yogi Bhajan. Small groups of people began to practice this form, and eventually the groups coalesced into an organization called 3HO.

3HO, which stands for "Happy, Healthy, Holy," has centers all over the United States. The people who live in these centers, or *ashrams,* maintain a lifestyle that is a uniquely American blend of traditional Sikh practices and Kundalini yoga techniques that are *not* part of traditional Sikhism. American Sikhs are vegetarians and they wear plain, white clothing, as well as white turbans. They also wear the traditional silver bangle on one wrist and, because they follow the Sikh rule against cutting the hair, the men often sport long beards. Practicing American Sikhs wake up very early in the morning to chant, recite from their holy book, and practice Kundalini yoga.

Kundalini yoga aims to awaken the kundalini, or serpentine energy, at the base of the spine. Once awakened, the kundalini progresses up the spine, making its way through the *chakras*—meaning "wheels"—of the body. As the kundalini progresses it burns away the karma of the practitioner. The goal is to move the kundalini all the way through the spine, through practices like yoga, and in this way experience full liberation.

Each of the chakras can be thought of as an energy center with particular qualities. As the kundalini travels up through the spine, it awakens each of these centers. The base, or root, chakra, located at the rectum, relates to our most basic instinct for survival. The next chakra, located in the genital area, relates to our sexuality. Further up, at the third chakra, which is located at the navel, we find the seat of our power and will. These lower centers give us a foundation for experiencing the centers above it, which are said to relate to our spirit and our higher potential. At the heart, where we experience feelings of love, is the fourth chakra. The throat, which is the fifth chakra, is the source of verbal communication. The sixth chakra, between the brows (also called the "third eye"), relates to our intuitive and psychic abilities. The seventh chakra, at the crown of the head, is called the seat of the soul. Finally, the eighth chakra goes beyond the body, to the aura.

A class usually begins with an invocation; then the postures and breathing practices begin. Fire breath, which is a rapid, rhythmic pumping of the diaphragm, is one of the most important breathing techniques used in this form of yoga. It is very easy to get dizzy or out of breath when first practicing this breath, or sometimes the hands and feet go numb and tingly; after awhile these symptoms pass. Practice of postures often involves the repetition of a movement. Often, this is done in conjunction with fire breath.

This is the sort of yoga that your body will feel instantly. It can be a bit like going for a run, and it can require and generate a lot of energy. The atmosphere of the class depends a lot on the teacher, though, and some teachers push their students, urging them to keep up, while others encourage students in a more gentle way.

If you go to a Kundalini class, there will almost certainly be chanting. This is where the devotional aspect of Kundalini yoga is most obvious, and some people are put off by it. But if you're at all inclined toward music or if you enjoy singing, you may find these chants very satisfying and soothing. If you are taking a class at an ashram, it's quite possible that a harmonium—a traditional Indian keyboard operated with a bellows—will be played along with the singing. These sweet melodies help to balance the intensity of the physical practice and they bring the mind to a more quiet, meditative place.

Kundalini yoga is a very powerful form, and it can be just the thing for many people. It's not as mainstream as other forms of yoga, but it is available through the ashrams where American Sikhs live, and sometimes there are classes offered outside of these communities. The communal aspect can in of itself be appealing to people who are looking for a community or who are perhaps curious about American Sikhs in particular.

Bikram Yoga

Bikram yoga gets its name from Bikram Choudhury, whose teacher was Bishnu Ghosh, the brother of Paramahansa Yogananda. Choudhury developed the Bikram system, and in the early '70s opened his first school in San Francisco. He is now based in Los Angeles, where he he is known by some as the "yogi of the stars." His school is called the Yoga College of India.

In Bikram yoga practice, the body's temperature is forced up by sealing off the room and turning the heat up high; this helps to warm muscles and flush toxins from the body. Bikram involves a set sequence of postures. There are twenty-six of these, and each one is usually practiced twice. Standing and balance poses come first, followed by back bends, forward bends, and twisting postures. Breathing is emphasized, and the ujjayi breath as well as fire breath are practiced. In a Bikram yoga class you use a mirror and are encourages to watch yourself; it's said that you are your own best teacher.

A Bikram yoga class makes for an intense workout and tends to attract men for that reason. However, Bikram yoga is meant to be open to everyone whatever your sex, age, or state of health. A certified Bikram yoga teacher should be able to help you pace yourself and make any necessary adaptions to postures.

Kripalu Yoga

Kripalu yoga is another branch of yoga that can be found in the West. In the United States, the best-known center for study of Kripalu yoga is in Massachusetts, where a large community has formed. This yoga retreat center boasts one of the bigger, more elaborate facilities, which can house about 15,000 guests a year. It is also thought to be one of the most beautiful retreat centers: it has been listed by *Newsweek* as the second most desirable hideaway in the country.

The community originally sprang up around a teacher, Amrit Desai, whose own teacher was a master of Kundalini yoga. At one point, Desai himself had a spontaneous kundalini awakening, and this led him to shift his teaching style to emphasize flow. His focus changed to helping people cultivate more sensitivity to the inner body as well as the outer body.

Students develop this inner attentiveness once they have learned the postures and can hold them for longer periods of time. At this stage, students are encouraged to follow the body's promptings and to sequence postures in a flowing, spontaneous way. This intuitive, creative approach makes Kripalu yoga appealing to some people. Kripalu is also attractive to those who want a gentler, slower-moving style—something that is in between restorative yoga and the other more vigorous forms of yoga.

Since its founding, the Kripalu community has undergone various changes over the years, the most notable being that Amrit Desai resigned in the 1990s over a sexual scandal. In spite of this fairly traumatic event, both the community and the yoga have survived. It's said that this community is the first to successfully transition from its original guru-disciple mode to a system that is more self-ruling.

Kripalu yoga's survival may be in part because it has not been a static form: it's been engaged in an ongoing growth process that has been unusually democratic, involving the combined efforts of its community. This interest in experimenting has led to another form called "Phoenix Rising Yoga Therapy."

Phoenix Rising Yoga Therapy

This form of yoga was developed by Michael Lee, a resident faculty member at Kripalu. It is a combination of bodywork and yoga and involves working one on one with a yoga therapist. It is not so much meant to address physical problems as to access the emotions through the body.

A session involves being supported by the therapist in various yoga postures. The client is encouraged to fully relax and release into each posture, allowing the therapist to offer full support. As the body becomes more deeply relaxed, emotions begin to bubble up to the surface. The idea is to consciously explore, release, and eventually integrate these feelings. The therapist facilitates this process by being a kind, loving presence and inviting dialogue when the client feels ready. The client always has the option to come out of a posture at any time.

Phoenix Rising Yoga Therapy is a safe and gentle form. Obviously, it's not for people who are looking for an intense workout. However, it may be useful to students of other yoga styles who experience difficult or painful emotions that can't be fully expressed or investigated in the context of a yoga class. Also, if you are especially interested in the emotional realm and know that you want to explore this area, Phoenix Rising Yoga Therapy may be a good style to work with.

Restorative Yoga

Most yoga classes include shavasana—or relaxation—at the end of class, after practicing postures that are active in nature. Restorative yoga is different in that it entirely eliminates the active postures and focuses instead on the relaxation part of yoga. It's geared toward people who are recovering from an injury or an illness or who just need to learn to de-stress. It can also be an appropriate form for older people.

Restorative yoga has been made more available to the general public in a book by Judith Lasater called *Relax and Renew: Restful Yoga for Stressful Times.* Restorative yoga, like Iyengar yoga, uses props—and, in fact, Lasater credits Iyengar for the development of many of its poses. Lasater has also drawn on her own experience as a yoga teacher, physical therapist, and mother to further refine this system.

Most of the poses are done lying on the floor, in various passive positions, with ample support from blankets and bolsters as well as other props. Like a regular yoga class, there is a logic in the sequencing of the poses. The poses are meant to bring the body into positions that invite and allow it—as well as the mind—to completely let go and relax. The poses are also designed to position the spine in different ways, sometimes curving it forward, backward, or twisting it. Also, Lasater recommends that an inverted pose be included in order to reverse the effects of gravity.

In these stressful times, everyone qualifies for restorative yoga. However, if you are in good health and are looking for a class that will challenge you physically, restorative yoga is not the route to go. It will nurture you but it won't actively build your strength. Also, the slow pacing of a typical restorative yoga class may not suit you. Nonetheless, this style can be a delicious way to de-stress. This sort of class can give you a complete experience while also teaching you a few very practical and simple things that you can do for yourself at home.

Tantra Yoga

Many people think of Tantra as the yoga of sex. Tantra did introduce ritualized sex, but this is only one aspect of Tantric practice, and it is not the basis of the system. Tantra is more about embracing all of life; it is sometimes called the "yoga of everything."

For the most part, Tantra yoga continues to be presented in the West primarily as sexual practices for partners. Though it is a distortion of the Tantric tradition, this Western version has enjoyed some success in the United States, and a number of people seem to have benefited from it. Charles and Caroline Muir are two of the most popular teachers. Margo Anand, author of *The Art of Sexual Ecstasy,* is also well known.

Tantra-based teaching in the United States is often in the format of seminars, usually for couples. Participants practice the Tantric attitude of embracing everything in themselves as well as in their partners. For heterosexual couples, this can mean that men learn to explore their feminine side, while women develop their masculine dimensions. Each person expands to include both the male and female polarities. Anand explains that when these polarities come together, a sacredness is felt and there is more of a sense of being connected to all of life.

Participants in seminars spend time looking at their habits and their blocks to intimacy. They work on increasing their capacity for intimacy and communication, as well learning specific techniques for prolonging and enhancing sexual pleasure.

Seminars do not usually involve nudity. The atmosphere is made as safe and comfortable for participants as possible.

A good place to start if you're interested in this kind of yoga is to read Anand's book, *The Art of Sexual Ecstasy*. If you're interested in knowing more about traditional Tantric, read Georg Feuerstein's *Tantra: The Path of Ecstasy*.

Yoga for Kids

As more adults discover the benefits of yoga, kids are being drawn to it, too. There are two different formats for these classes: classes are either for children only, or for children and their parents.

Children are often naturals at yoga. They are generally more energetic and limber than adults, and yoga can seem easy and fun for them. Often, though, they don't have the same capacity for concentration, so they usually respond best to more vigorous forms of yoga in which there is continuous movement and physical challenge. They also appreciate a playful approach, and can be great fun for a teacher. The teacher, however, must be skilled at working with kids; the success of the class really rests with his or her ability to reach the students.

The benefits that children experience are the same as those for adults: they become stronger, more flexible (and there are a few children who start out being surprisingly inflexible), and they learn to concentrate their attention more completely. Some parents feel that yoga is helpful in correcting behavioral problems, too. Classes that include parents provide a new way for parents and children to interact and bond.

Although classes for kids are harder to find, they do exist; yoga studios occasionally offer them; your local YMCA might also be a good place to look. There are also a few good books available, including one by Mary Stewart called *Yoga for Children*.

Yoga for the Elderly

Yoga is for older adults, too. It is never too late to start. The late Vanda Scaravelli, a famous yoga teacher who was based in Italy, began her study of yoga in her forties and for many years proved the age-defying benefits of regular yoga practice. There are some very inspiring pictures of Vanda in yoga postures that many younger people can't perform.

Some of the most obvious features of aging are a general loss of flexibility and strength and a tightening up of the spine and back. With careful, deliberate, and regular yoga practice, flexibility and strength can gradually be restored. The body—even in old age—is surprisingly resilient and responsive when given the proper attention.

A restorative yoga class might be an appropriate place to start for some seniors. But for many older adults, getting down on the floor is awkward and uncomfortable—at least at first— and in yoga classes that cater specifically to the elderly, liberal use is made of chairs. You might be surprised how creatively chairs, as well as other props, like windowsills and walls, can be used. Almost any yoga posture can be adapted in some way to the needs and the limitations of the elderly practitioner.

Classes for older people are less common in yoga studios; a good place to look for one is at a YMCA or senior center.

Yoga for the Disabled

I have had the good fortune to work with a number of disabled people, mostly people with cerebral palsy or multiple sclerosis, in my yoga classes. Cerebral palsy affects the nervous system and can range from a mild condition to a very severe condition in which there is no consistent muscular control over the body; even speech is impossible.

I had one student for a time who had a less severe case of cerebral palsy and was able to walk, albeit in a halting, somewhat haphazard manner. She came to my classes and was able to do all of the postures, in her own way. It was extremely moving to see her standing in warrior pose, or some other asana, bravely holding it as steadily as she could, while her hand waved wildly in front of her body, like a fish wending its way through water. Another student came for awhile in her wheelchair and managed to flop herself down onto the floor before each class, where she worked the entire class, making many adaptations to suit her body's capacities.

Both of these students received something by being in class and working with their bodies and their minds, from moment to moment, like any other student. These students were also very important to the atmosphere of the class, though they may not have realized it: they inspired other students and reminded us all of many things. They were especially a reminder of the need to not be so attached to and identified with this body we are given: we are more than the body.

If you have a serious physical disability and want to take a yoga class, you might be able to take a regular class: it depends on you, your situation, and the teacher. Any good teacher will welcome your interest in yoga, but not every teacher will be skilled at integrating you into the class. If the class is really large, for instance, the teacher simply might not have time to help you out with each new posture or movement. If you feel comfortable and confident working out your own adaptations, you may be very happy in such a class. It may be more satisfying, though, to have more guidance and a class that is designed specifically to meet your needs. These classes are becoming more common in hospitals. Like anyone, you will have to find the right teacher.

FINDING A TEACHER

It's important to have a teacher when you first start practicing yoga. Some people are tempted to just get a video or two and learn that way—and there are many wonderful, comprehensive videos to choose from—but there is no substitute for a teacher.

A teacher can give guidance that you can't possible glean from a video, and this guidance will make yoga a safe activity for you. Through a teacher you will learn how to do the postures (asanas), the breathing exercises (pranayama), and the relaxation (shavasana) correctly. Your teacher can also help you understand your ingrained, unconscious habits: if you are a person who drives yourself and tries too hard, a good teacher will recognize that and encourage you to ease up and relax more. Or if you are a little lethargic and heavy in your practice, a teacher can help to energize you. Once you have studied for a while, and have some sense of what it is you are doing, then, if you want to learn from videos, by all means do so.

How you come to yoga—or how yoga comes to you—is a mysterious process. Chance alone—or fate—can bring you to a teacher. Or you can approach the business of finding a teacher with some method. If you have a sense of what style yoga you might like to pursue, that will give you some direction. Maybe you have mild curiosity and you want to start out with a small dose of *some* kind of yoga, but you don't really know which. Whatever your level of interest, there is a teacher—maybe several teachers—for you.

In India, great respect is accorded a teacher or guru, and traditionally, a true seeker offers himself, entrusts his life, to the teacher. What the teacher offers to those who want it is wisdom—guidance along the path to enlightenment—and the student must have a level of depth, seriousness, and commitment in order to even be accepted by the teacher. Sometimes a teacher will appear disinterested, or be inaccessible for a time, in order to test the student's sincerity. Once a student is accepted and initiated as a disciple by the teacher, they enter a relationship that can be much closer than what many Westerners are used to. There is a passion and sacredness in their contract, and this bond can last for a lifetime. There are many very interesting books that throw light on the teacher-disciple relationship, including *Autobiography of a Yogi* by Paramahansa Yogananda, and T. K. V. Desikachar's book, *Health, Healing and Beyond*.

Westerners often approach teachers with a different set of expectations. It is very common—at least in the beginning—for people to be more casual, to pick and choose, just taking a class or two here and there, and then decide on a teacher. Students do not necessarily develop any sort of personal relationship with a teacher, nor is there any particular commitment on the part of the student. The tendency in the West is for teachers to maintain a certain distance from their students, so while they may be guides in the yoga studio, they are not necessarily involved in a student's day-to-day life or decision-making processes. This seems to suit the temperament of Westerners, who generally value their privacy and independence. But some students may yearn for more spiritual guidance and seek out a closer, disciple-like relationship.

This is available to those who want it, but requires a teacher who is willing and able to meet a student on that level; it may take more time to find such a teacher.

One of the best ways to look for a teacher is to start asking around. Find out if any of your friends are doing yoga and what they think of the classes they've taken. Listen to what people are saying about different teachers and then, if what you hear is appealing, go see for yourself.

It is impossible for any one teacher to please everyone who comes to a class; teachers have their own particular personalities and develop individual teaching styles. So, while a certain teacher may suit one student, he or she doesn't always match the needs of another. That's why it's worth looking around for a teacher you like. You may want to attend several classes taught by different people. You may also want to take a few classes with the same teacher; sometimes a teacher can grow on you. See how you feel in each class, and trust your inner response. A few things to consider that may be helpful:

- Does the teacher show respect for you and others?

- Do you feel at ease with the teacher?

- Does the teacher inspire you?

- Does the teacher seem kind and caring? (Some teachers may seem more serious—perhaps even severe at times—but this attitude does not have to mean they are uncaring. There are teachers who use the "tough love" approach, and some people respond well to this style.)

- Do you feel your questions are welcomed? Is the teacher accessible?

- Are your questions answered?

- Does the teacher give clear verbal and visual instruction?

- Does the teacher's physical touch feel appropriate and impart useful information? (Some teachers ask for permission before giving physical adjustments, but this is not by any means the norm.)

- How much experience does a teacher have? (Don't be too quick to dismiss a teacher who hasn't taught for a long time: he or she may have something to offer you. Likewise, a teacher who's very experienced isn't by default the best choice for you.)

- Does the teacher give you the attention and feedback you feel you need?

- Does the teacher radiate qualities you would like to cultivate more in yourself?

- What's the general atmosphere of the class? Is it one you feel good in? Do you like the feeling of the group as a whole?

- Do you like the physical space in which the class is taking place? (A studio doesn't have to be fancy to be a good place to learn yoga. What's more important is that it be warm enough and clean. Good light is nice to have, too.)

- How do you feel after the class? (You may feel like you've worked, but you should feel good. You should feel better than when you first walked in.)

There is a saying that when the student is ready, the teacher will appear. It could be that you will find one teacher to study with for a while, and then something draws you to another. Many people study with more than one teacher at a time. This can sometimes be confusing, as there can be a great deal of variety and difference in what's being taught and how it's being presented, but it's also quite possible to learn and draw from multiple sources. Sometimes, as we start out we don't really know what we're looking for, but as we gain experience it becomes more clear what we really want and need. Also, as we proceed, our needs may change and lead us to a different teacher.

What You Owe the Teacher

If you are attending a yoga class for the very first time, or even if you're relatively new to yoga, please tell your teacher. Definitely let your teacher know about any injuries, limitations, or physical conditions (including pregnancy). Feel free to voice any general concerns that you may have—*before* you begin class. If you are someone who has suffered abuse—sexual or other-wise—and you don't feel comfortable being physically adjusted or doing partner work, inform the teacher. It's very important for teachers to know about these things, and there is no way for them to know without students telling them. If you have a serious condition, it may not be appropriate for you to do yoga at all; it's a good idea in such a case to consult with a doctor first, before you begin a yoga practice.

Always be sensible about your physical limitations. If you feel you may be injuring yourself by practicing a particular asana or movement, don't do it. It is much wiser to be respectful of your limitations than to get overly enthusiastic and hurt yourself. Also, there are often adaptations that can be made to postures, and a teacher can help you with these if you request help.

Some teachers have guidelines that must be honored if you are going to study with them. So, for instance, a teacher may request that you wear particular clothing, like tights or shorts, which make the musculature of the body more plain and visible, so the teacher can see clearly what you are doing.

If something about the class really isn't working for you, let the teacher know about your experience. Perhaps the class is too advanced, and the teacher can recommend another class or teacher instead. Especially if you need to leave the class before it's over, let the teacher know why; it can be very disconcerting for a teacher to have a student disappear with no explanation.

Likewise, if you really like something about the class, teachers always appreciate hearing positive feedback. Sometimes students are shy about taking up a teacher's time; don't be if you really have something important to say. Teachers don't always know how deeply their students are being affected, and it's good for them to be told.

PRACTICING ON YOUR OWN

After you've been studying yoga for a while and you've been feeling the benefits of your practice, you may be inspired to start doing yoga on your own. Daily practice is recommended, and it's exciting to find yourself moving into this stage.

The first thing to do is to locate, or create, a place in which to practice. Clear the room enough to have space to move around in freely. You don't want to be breathing in lots of dust as you practice, so make sure the room is clean. Adjust the room's temperature so that it's warm enough to practice in comfortably. (It's not advised to practice in a cold room, and it won't feel good, either.) If the room is quiet, so much the better. Some people like to make an altar space on which to place flowers, incense, or a picture of a teacher. Do whatever you need to do to make the room appealing, so that you will want to be in it.

You will probably want to buy yourself a sticky mat, and if you are used to using other props like straps, blocks, or blankets, then invest in those, too. Some people also like to have a stop-watch or clock so that poses can be timed.

Then find a time to go into your room and practice. If you can, get up before the sun and practice in the early morning hours: this is a quiet time, and you will benefit from starting your day with yoga. For some people, though, this is not practical. Find a time that works for you. If possible, set aside roughly the same time of day for yourself: this will help get your body and mind into the habit of practice. Again, though, this is not always possible, so be flexible. After all, in doing yoga, you are trying to cultivate flexibility not just in your body, but in your whole life. If the demands of your life prevent you from doing as thorough and long a practice as you might like, do what you can. Never tell yourself, "It's all or nothing": twenty minutes of yoga is much better than no yoga.

Some people like to use videos or audiotapes to guide them through a practice session. These are wonderful tools after you've had some experience with yoga but aren't sure yet how to proceed on your own. You know that you want to practice, and you have some proficiency in the poses, but you don't really know how to sequence the poses yourself. Try a video or tape for a while—try several if you want to, because there are many to choose from and they vary quite a bit—and when you feel ready, start experimenting on your own.

This can be a scary transition for some people, but it's worth trying. You might want to take notes after a class some time, and see if you can practice from those. Or just get down on the floor and see what you can remember. It may be helpful to try to conjure your teacher's voice into your mind, hearing that voice guiding you. See what your body and your mind tell you. You probably know more than you think.

Always end your session with shavasana.

And finally, the way a yoga practice typically finishes is by sitting comfortably, joining the palms, and bowing to the teacher. We say, *"Namaste,"* as we do this, which is a traditional greeting. It means, "I bow to the divine within you." You can do this as you finish your own private practice as well. It's good to have a clear beginning and end. You can also think of it as a way of bowing to the teacher in yourself, the Self.

six

YOGA FOR WOMEN

Most of the known yoga texts indicate that yoga was traditionally a male practice. It's possible that women in ancient times practiced yoga, too—and they may have made some contributions to its development. But now is when the influence of women is most obvious. Within this century, the tables have turned and most yoga classes—at least in the West—contain a greater number of women than men. As a result of this shift in the practicing population, yoga has had to change to accommodate the needs of women, whose biology is profoundly different from men's.

This biological difference is most apparent once a girl has reached puberty and begins menstruating. From this point on, the monthly hormonal cycle is a part of her life. For a few girls and women, this cycle is not particularly remarkable. It's safe to say, though, that the majority of women are aware of their menstrual cycles, and quite a few are impacted in negative ways. Symptoms range from mild to extreme. Some women have only a little discomfort and can function no matter where they are during their cycle; others have such severe symptoms that they are put completely out of commission for several days. It's not uncommon for women to experience premenstrual syndrome (PMS) at some point in their lives.

The menstrual system is regulated by delicate hormonal shifts in the body. If the hormones are unbalanced, this can result in painful, or uncomfortable, side-effects. Because yoga can work at the level of the glandular system, over time it can help create more balanced hormonal activity. In addition, yoga makes practitioners more sensitive and, as a result, helpful dietary changes may come more easily. Caffeine, alcohol, and sugar are the main culprits in PMS. If you've been practicing yoga for awhile, you may find that you have less craving for these substances.

Certain yoga postures can be especially helpful for relieving painful menstrual symptoms. Lower back pain, for instance, can be relieved by lying on the back with the knees drawn into the chest. Resting the legs at a wall can counteract excess water retention. Back-arching postures sometimes help relieve cramping.

Pregnancy and birth are of course an important part of many women's lives. It makes sense, then, that prenatal yoga has become so popular: it's clearly needed. Likewise, because women often spend a number of years raising their children, they have special needs that are most readily addressed in postpartum yoga classes. Menopause is another turning point in women's lives, and this passage can be made more smooth by yoga practice. This last is an area of yoga that has not been sufficiently developed. No doubt in years to come we will see more classes geared specifically to women in menopause. For now, if you are taking yoga classes during menopause and you're experiencing troublesome symptoms, it may be useful to let your teacher know. Particularly if your teacher is a woman who has gone through this stage, she may have some helpful suggestions.

PRENATAL YOGA

Before yoga became popularized in the West, Krishnamacharya had begun encouraging women, and pregnant women in particular, to practice yoga. This came about through his discovery of an ancient yoga text known as the *Yoga Rahasaya*. According to Desikachar, "No other Yoga text places such emphasis upon the importance of considering the uniqueness of the individual in prescribing practice—including such characteristics as age, sex, body type, and station in life. There is also a great deal of emphasis upon the need for, and the nature of, Yogic practice for pregnant women." Desikachar also makes a point of saying that his father eventually came to view women as actually being the more reliable transmitters of yoga.

It is now becoming much more commonplace to see yoga classes offered to pregnant women. There are many women who feel that yoga has been tremendously helpful both during pregnancy and while going through labor and delivery.

A few women go through pregnancy with great ease. For many others, the experience can be more mixed and shifting hormones, along with a swelling belly, can be traumatizing, uncomfortable, and unpleasant at times. All these changes can be overwhelming. Yoga can restore a sense of control by offering some practical ways to cope with these changes.

On the physical level, the proper practice of prenatal yoga can cultivate strength and endurance, which are critical not just for labor and delivery but also after the baby has arrived. (Many women become so focused on the hurdle of giving birth that they forget how much energy they'll need for healing themselves later and taking care of an infant.) Prenatal yoga can also encourage a gentle and gradual widening of the hips in preparation for birth. Postural problems can be addressed, and sometimes lower back pain—which most pregnant women experience at some stage—can be alleviated. Symptoms of sciatica are sometimes relieved, too. In addition, the upper body can be made stronger to support the growing weight of the breasts and to make it easier later on to carry a baby and to nurse without strain.

Prenatal yoga classes are often less rigorous than other classes. They strengthen a woman's body but in a gentle way. If available, props are frequently used to give a little extra support to the body in certain poses. Poses need to be modified or avoided entirely depending on the stage of pregnancy a woman is in. So, for instance, after the third or fourth month, postures are not done while lying on the back: once the fetus has grown to a certain size, a back-lying position can impede the return flow of blood to the mother's heart. Also, a pregnant woman has to be careful not to overstretch, as her muscles and ligaments are already loosening up on their own, due to the secretion of the hormone relaxin.

Prenatal yoga classes often work more specifically with the breath, as this is a particularly useful tool for the laboring woman. Also, more time is usually devoted to relaxation. Being pregnant is a lot of work and it's appropriate to rest more during pregnancy. But it's also important to learn to relax into the actual process of pregnancy. The body has an intuitive, instinctual wisdom that takes over at conception. What's needed is to trust this, and relax enough to allow the process to unfold. This is especially true as a woman goes in to labor: she must learn to release, soften, and open her body so that the baby can emerge. Yoga techniques for relaxation can be extremely helpful in this respect.

Yoga practice also creates a space in which a woman can contemplate more generally what it is to carry and bring forth life—to be engaged in this astonishing project of making something from nothing. Pregnancy and birth are utterly natural— and at the same time miraculous. This passage puts a woman directly in touch with a creative source that is both of her and beyond her.

If you are inexperienced in yoga and you are pregnant, it's a good idea to seek out a prenatal class. Such a class will be more geared to your specific needs and you will have the comfort of being among other women who are going through the same experience. If you happen to attend a regular yoga class while you are pregnant, let your teacher know—especially if it's not obvious! Also, it's a good idea to err on the side of caution and check in with your doctor about what sort of exercise is appropriate, especially when considering any sort of new exercise program.

POSTPARTUM YOGA

Pregnancy, childbirth, and early motherhood are extremely physical and require a great deal of energy that new mothers sometimes feel they don't have. In addition, there can be some new physical challenges with this terrain.

Most new mothers complain about neck and shoulder discomfort. These symptoms are a natural result of the new load you're carrying: not only are you bending over and holding your baby for many hours a day, you're also carrying all of the paraphernalia that comes with a baby—car seat, diaper bag, and so on.

Fortunately, many yoga postures can help you heal your body and make adjustments to your new life. Even a few minutes of the most basic stretches can be restorative and you can learn these in the context of a postpartum class. A regular class might work, too, though it's not likely to address your needs as directly as a postpartum class would. Plus, you'll probably need to be with your baby, and a sensible postpartum yoga class welcomes babies.

Babies are indeed a big part of the atmosphere. While prenatal yoga classes can be calm and meditative, postpartum classes usually veer in the other direction: they can be chaotic and wild at times, depending on what sort of mood the babies are in. These classes are also a lot of fun and offer a nurturing environment for women who might otherwise be trying to cope on their own.

seven

A GOOD BASIC ROUTINE

If you are curious to try a few yoga postures on your own before investigating a class, you'll find the following sequence helpful. Even just looking at the pictures will give you some idea of what yoga postures are about—at least externally. You'll also get a sense of how a sequence of postures might be put together.

Because it can be confusing to follow instructions from a book, you may want to try this sequence out with a friend, reading the instructions to each other. You may also want to reread the chapter on Principles of Yoga Practice. Here are a few other guidelines:

- Find a clean, warm, spacious place where you can move around freely.

- Have an empty stomach. It's generally recommended that you practice three or four hours after a meal. Sometimes a light snack can be taken an hour or so before you practice.

- Yoga is done with bare feet. This allows you to be more aware of how your feet are working. It also keeps you from slipping in the standing poses.

- Don't do anything that doesn't feel right. If you are pregnant or have an injury, you may want to just read this chapter without actually trying it out. Consult a doctor, then take a class that teaches these poses, and use this chapter as a reminder for a daily routine.

- Come into each position slowly. Hold it for a few breaths. Come out of it slowly. Give yourself ample time to rest in between postures, letting your mind register the effects on your system.

1 MEDITATION

It's very helpful to start your practice with meditation; doing this will help bring your attention more fully to your actions. When you meditate, you should be in a comfortable position. If you can sit cross-legged, seat yourself on the folded edge of a blanket, giving your lumbar spine (lower back) plenty of support. A general principle to keep in mind when you sit this way is that the knees should not be higher than the hips; if they are, your back will be stressed, and it will be impossible to relax. If you need more support, sit on several blankets or get yourself a *zafu* (meditation pillow). If it's impossible for you to sit comfortably in a cross-legged position on the floor, with your knees at least as low as your hips, sit on a chair instead, drawing yourself toward the edge of the chair to discourage your spine from slumping.

If you're not used to meditating, you don't have to sit for a long time: three or four minutes can do wonders for stilling the mind. See if you can notice the quality of your mental state. Are you agitated, thinking lots of thoughts at once? Or are you feeling tired and dull? Start by just noticing your mind's state, without trying to change it.

How does your body feel? Do you feel strong and centered? Do you have aches or pains anywhere? Notice how your body feels. Some people feel that once they start meditation they must sit rigidly in one position. This is counterproductive. If you're not quite comfortable, shift your position slightly. Take a moment also to note which specific areas of the body may need more care and attention, so that you can be more conscious of them once you start to move.

Then turn your attention to your breath. What's the quality of the breath? Is it deep? Shallow and contained? One of the most calming things for an agitated mind is to focus on the breath, inviting it to deepen. Taking deep breaths can also energize a tired, dull mind. If you find it hard to keep your mind focused on the quality of your breath, try just counting breaths. If you count backward, starting at thirty, this will keep your mind more alert. After you have spent a few minutes meditating, then try out the postures.

This movement provides a good way to prepare and warm up your body for more active poses; it gently loosens the whole spine and also strengthens and energizes the arms and wrists.

Get down on all fours. Adjust your hands so that they're directly beneath your shoulders, and bring your knees so that they are underneath your hips. Let your back round, so that the mid-back lifts toward the ceiling. Draw your head down, allowing its full weight to drop. This will help the back of the neck to release. Hold this position for a few breaths.

Then move your spine the other way, so that you sway your back. The belly drops down toward the floor, and your head lifts up. Be attentive to how your back feels, and if it seems like too much sway, then neutralize your back a little. Observe how your neck and throat feel as well. If there's tension anywhere in these areas, adjust your head a little differently. Hold this position for a few breaths. See if you can hold here without sagging your shoulders.

Then try going back and forth between these two positions, coordinating this movement with your breath. What's most natural is to breathe in as your chest becomes more expansive: this is the Dog-Tilt position. As you breathe out, curve your spine into Cat Stretch. See if the movement can be fluid and energetic at the same time. If it bothers your wrists to be on all fours, try supporting yourself on your forearms instead.

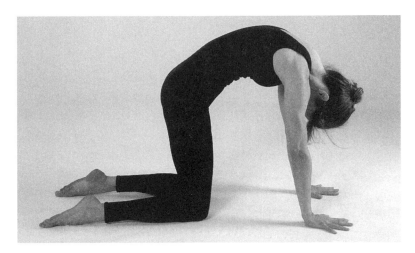

Cat Stretch

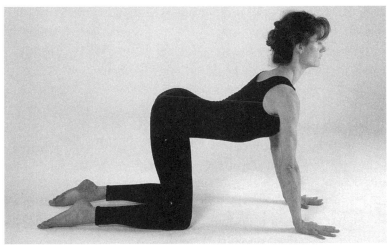

Dog Tilt

3 CHILD'S POSE

This position lengthens the spine and gives relief to the lower back. It allows the shoulder blades to release away from the spine. It can also help to loosen and open up the hip joints.

From the position on all fours, let your weight sink back so that you rest the buttocks onto the heels. Drop your head down, resting your forehead on the floor. Bring the arms alongside the body, or, if that's awkward, stack one arm on top of the other in front of you, and rest your forehead there. To get comfortable, you can shift the hips and knees around, playing with how wide apart your knees are. The main thing is to find a position that allows you to rest. If it's painful to your knees or hips, don't force yourself. It may work to slip a pillow over your calves and rest that way. If that still doesn't work, try keeping your hips higher off the heels, or try lying on your back and drawing the knees into the chest (see photo of Rocking on the Spine, page 125).

4 DOWNWARD-FACING DOG

Downward-facing dog is a very strengthening and energizing pose; it is one of the central poses of many yoga systems. It builds strength in the arms and back and also cultivates more mobility in the spine and pelvis. The backs of the legs, particularly the hamstrings, are stretched as well.

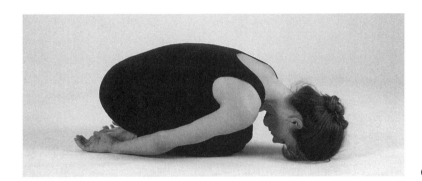

Child's Pose

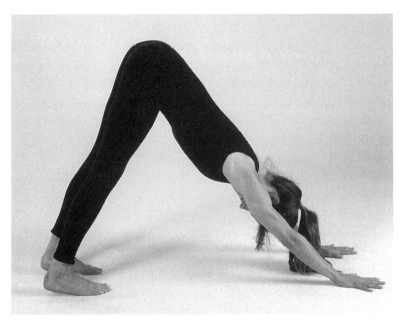

Downward-Facing
Dog

Get down on all fours again. Align your hands under your shoulders and your knees beneath your hips. Curl your toes under and slowly lift your knees off the floor. Bring your body to an inverted V. The hips lift up, with the back lengthening. At the same time, the heels sink downward toward the floor.

Don't look forward: make sure that the back of the neck is relaxed.

If you find that the backs of the legs are extremely tight, allow the knees to bend a little. Once you've had a little practice, this position will feel easier, and you can work on lengthening the legs.

Hold this position for several deep breaths. Then come back down to Child's Pose—or some variation—and rest for a few breaths. (Again, if Child's Pose is not comfortable, you can rest on your back with your knees drawn in toward your chest.)

5 TADASANA, MOUNTAIN POSE

This is a basic pose in yoga. It helps you be more generally aware of your posture. You'll also be more conscious of your feet and how you use them. In this pose you'll have a taste of the concentration and solidity that's possible in balance poses.

In this pose, you come to a standing position, joining your feet and placing your weight evenly on your feet. Try to be solid

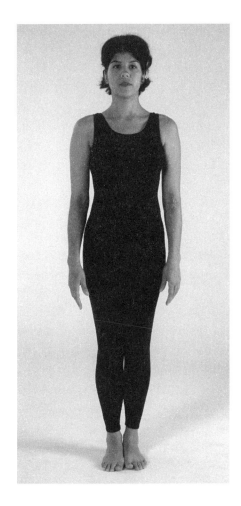

Tadasana,
Mountain Pose

and firm, like a mountain. Try not to overemphasize the weight in your heels or the balls of the feet. Stand straight, without being rigid, so that your shoulders don't slump forward. Then gently tighten your thighs so that the kneecaps lift slightly upward. Avoid locking your knees.

Hold this position, focusing on your breath. Try a variation, with both arms extending upward.

6 TREE POSE

Tree Pose is a balance pose. It will strengthen your legs, especially the ankles, and it will improve your concentration and focus.

From Mountain Pose, slowly shift your weight into one leg. Bend the opposite knee, drawing the foot high up onto the thigh. Press your foot slightly into the thigh to stabilize it. Turn the knee outward, to the side. Bring your palms together at the heart. See if you can balance there. If your balance is unsteady, keep trying. If you have your balance, try extending the arms up overhead.

Hold for a few breaths. Then release your leg slowly. Shake your legs out a little bit and take a few breaths in Mountain Pose before you try the other side.

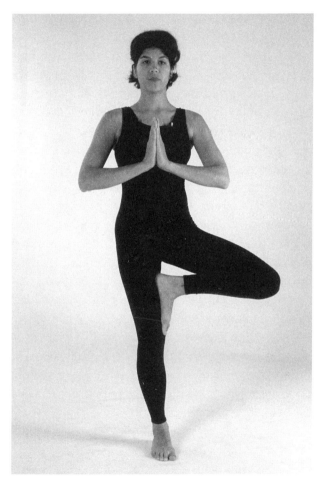

Tree Pose

In this pose, you'll strengthen and lengthen the legs. The hips will become more open. You'll also increase your neck's range of motion, open the chest, and increase your capacity for balance.

Take a wide stance, with the feet several feet apart, and turn your right foot about 90 degrees to the right. Turn the left foot in as well, but not quite as sharply. Firm the thighs without locking your knees. Extend the arms out to the sides, and reach toward the right. Let the right hand come down onto your right leg—anywhere *above* or *below* the kneecap—and extend the left arm straight up toward the ceiling. Try to align your upper body so that it extends over your right leg, instead of tipping forward. Turn your gaze upward if your neck can do this without straining. If the neck strains here, then try a different head position, just looking forward or down instead.

Hold for a few breaths. Imagine the arms and legs growing away from the trunk of the body. Slowly come back up, and turn your feet the other way to do the other side.

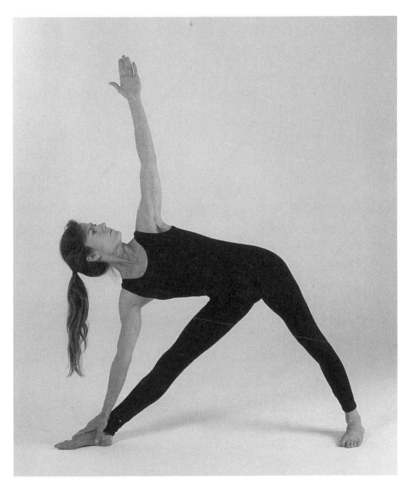

Triangle Pose

This pose lengthens the backs of the legs. As the legs become more flexible, the back and neck will also begin to stretch. It also compresses the abdominal area so that the internal organs press against each other, effectively massaging one another.

Start with the feet in Mountain Pose. Extend the arms out to the sides. Then slowly hinge at the hips, extending the trunk of the body forward. Try to keep the back long and extended as you come forward. Slowly fold down toward the legs. You can start by just letting the upper body hang. The arms can dangle, or you can clasp your elbows. Let you head drop so there's no tension in the back of the neck.

If the back of your legs feel very tight, allow the knees to bend a little. Also, if your back is weak, instead of folding forward into the position, you can roll your spine downward with knees bent. This action will be easier on your back.

Hold the forward bend for a few breaths. When you're ready, bend your knees and roll back up to standing.

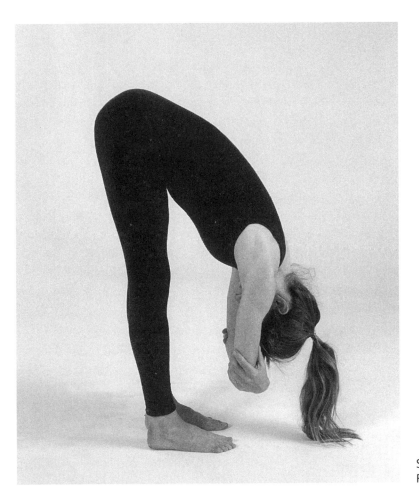

Standing
Forward Bend

9 WARRIOR POSE

Warrior Pose is a strengthening pose, particularly for the legs, but also for the arms. It will open up the hips and widen the chest. It will cultivate your endurance while at the same time flushing your body with energy.

Take a wide stance and turn your feet to the right again, as you did for Triangle Pose. Extend the arms out to the sides, to the height of the shoulders. Bend your right knee and line it up directly over your right ankle. Turn your gaze out over your right hand.

Hold this position for a few breaths. Extend out through the arms as you hold here, and let the chest open wide. Try not to lean out over your right leg; keep the spine upright instead.

Come back up, relaxing the arms. Turn your feet the other way and do the same thing on the left side.

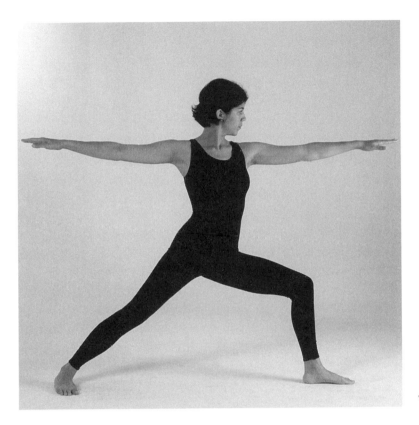

Warrior Pose

10 SEATED FORWARD BEND

Like the Standing Forward Bend, this pose invites more length and flexibility into the backs of the legs. It will also lengthen the back. If you come far enough forward, the pose will create a gentle massaging of the internal organs.

Sit on the floor with your legs extended forward. Flex the feet, energizing your legs so that there's a feeling of extending the legs through the heels. Press the backs of the legs down toward the floor. Lift the spine to sit upright.

Extend your arms overhead and hold for a few breaths. Then slowly extend forward toward your legs. Rather than rounding your back, see if you can lengthen it. Let your arms rest on your legs wherever they can reach, or catch hold of the feet if you can reach that far.

Hold for a few breaths, keeping your legs energetic if you can. If this is very awkward, try relaxing the legs and just letting the upper body droop forward. This is a more passive approach to the pose that can also be beneficial.

11 ROCKING ON THE SPINE

This is a good way to release the lower back, and makes a good alternative to Child's Pose if that pose is too difficult.

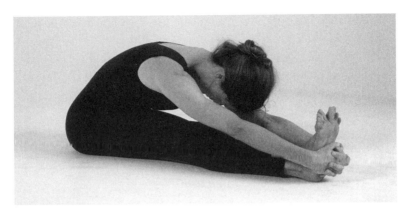

Seated
Forward Bend

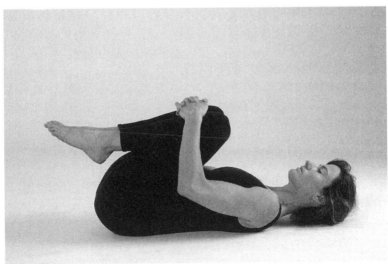

Rocking on
the Spine

Lie on your back and draw your knees toward your chest, holding them stable. You can just hold this position, or you can rock on the spine from side to side or front to back.

12 SPINAL TWIST

This pose creates more mobility in the spine and often feels especially good in the lower back. It is a chest- and shoulder-opening posture and, like the Seated and Standing Forward Bends, creates some massage-like action in the internal organs.

From the previous position, with the knees drawn into the chest, let the arms come out to the sides, to a T. Slowly drop your knees over to one side, letting them rest all the way onto the floor. You can look straight up toward the ceiling, or if your neck permits it, look away from your knees.

If this position creates too much twist for your spine, try placing a pillow beneath your legs, so that your legs don't have to drop down so far. This will reduce the twist in your spine.

Hold for several long, slow breaths, just resting and letting gravity do the work. This is a passive pose. Then bring your knees back up, rest in this position for a few breaths, and drop the knees over to the other side.

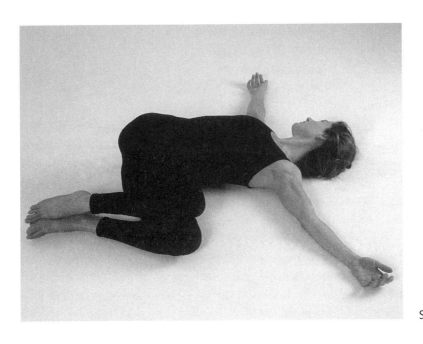

Spinal Twist

13 SHAVASANA, RELAXATION

Relaxation comes after asana practice for good reason. For one thing, we're often somewhat tired after practice and this makes it easier to relax. The mind is also in a more receptive state at this point, because its movements have been somewhat stilled through focus on physical activity. Relaxation becomes more natural over time and leads gradually into a stronger connection with your essential nature. Experiences of deep relaxation help prepare for the next stage, pranayama, which takes us further into our practice of stilling and focusing the mind.

Stretch yourself out on your back. Separate the feet slightly. Let the arms rest loosely at your sides, with the palms turned up if that's comfortable. If your lower back needs extra support, roll a blanket or a pillow and place it under the knees. This bending of your knees will let the lower back flatten a little more and may help you feel more at ease.

As you lie here, relax. Let the weight of your body drop into the floor. Give all of your cares and worries to the Earth. Let go of everything, just for a few minutes. Keep scanning your body, noticing if there's any residual tension. When you find areas that are still holding, release them. As you relax your body more and more with each breath, keep some part of your awareness on the sensations that arise as you rest.

If this is too abstract, try counting your breaths. Start at fifty, or forty, and count backward. Notice if your mind strays and pick up where you left off. Sometimes this technique can help settle the mind; then it's more possible to pay closer attention to relaxing your body.

See if you can stay here for ten minutes. If that's too long, start out with five, or even three minutes, and gradually increase the length of time.

Variations on Shavasana

1 If you have trouble lying still, or if you have trouble even knowing what it means to relax, then try doing the opposite: try creating tension in your body, and then relaxing. You can do this by consciously gripping each muscle in your body—including the muscles in your face—all at the same time. Tighten everything as firmly as possible, and hold this tension for a few seconds. Then release, and see how it feels. Repeat this a few times, and then see if you can lie still for a few minutes.

2 Another way to do this is to progressively tighten and release individual muscle groups. You start at the feet and work your way upward. Try gripping your toes and holding for a few seconds, and then releasing for a few breaths. Feel the muscles in your toes relaxing. Then engage the muscles of your feet, pressing your toes away from you in a pointed position. Hold for a few seconds, then release, again observing the tension as it drains away from your feet. Flex your

feet so that you're tightening your calf muscles, holding this position for a few breaths, and releasing. Continue up the body in this fashion, working your way all the way up to the crown of your head.

3 Some people find it helpful to imagine light moving through the body. Again, you can do this by focusing the light in your feet and slowly moving it up through your body. Or you can progress from the head down toward the toes. Once you've covered the whole body, you can imagine the light spreading into the space around your body.

The point is to be able to find a way to relax. If this is especially challenging for you in the beginning, be creative and experiment until you find what works. Your efforts will pay off, and you'll find over time that you will be able to drop into this quiet space with more and more ease.

PRACTICING PRANAYAMA

You may want to try the above sequence of postures a few times. After you've worked with this routine, you might want to get a taste of pranayama practice. Make sure that you do pranayama after asana practice, and that you give yourself a little time *between* shavasana and pranayama—at least fifteen minutes.

In pranayama, the goal is to immerse ourselves completely in awareness of the breath. Because this is easier said than done, we use certain techniques for focusing our attention. These involve breaking the breath down into its parts: the inhale and exhale. As with asana practice, we can do different things with these parts of the breath: we can balance them equally, or give more time to the exhalation than the inhalation (the exhalation is emphasized in pranayama). We can hold the breath in for a certain amount of time, or we can hold the breath out.

One big difference between pranayama and asana practice is that pranayama is done in a simple seated position, without moving. For that reason, it's critical that we be comfortable. If we become uncomfortable as we're practicing, then we'll lose our awareness of the breath. So it's important first to find a position in which the body will not distract us. As with meditation, this can mean sitting on the edge of a blanket on the floor, sitting on a zafu, or sitting in a chair.

A Few Breathing Exercises

Here are some general principles to follow when working with breathing exercises. Avoid forcing anything. For instance, if you have a cold and your nostrils are blocked, then you don't want to breathe in through the nose. Also, if you have problems with your eyes (glaucoma, for instance) or ears, or if you are pregnant, don't hold your breath. The same applies for people with blood pressure problems or heart problems. Stop if your breath gets irregular. Also stop if you start to feel dizzy. Finally, once you have finished your exercises, always rest in shavasana for five or ten minutes.

The ujjayi breath is a good place to start. This involves slightly closing the throat so that the breath makes an audible sound as it moves in and out. Let the breath be expansive and steady. It may take some getting used to at first, but once you've practiced for a while, you'll find that the ujjayi breath comes more automatically. Once you've become familiar and comfortable with this way of breathing, there are some other ways to work with the breath that will serve as an introduction to the more precise yogic breathing techniques.

- *Alternate nostril breathing.* Sitting in a comfortable position, bring your right hand up to your nose. The thumb is used to control the opening of the right nostril, while the ring and pinky fingers control the opening of the left nostril. Start by blocking the left nostril and taking a full, even breath through the right nostril. Then block the right nostril with the thumb, and unblock the left nostril, slowly letting the air out of the left nostril. Repeat the same thing, this time taking the inhale through the left side, and letting it out through the right. This makes a complete cycle. You can try eight or ten cycles of this at a time. Keep the breath even and deep. Lie down and rest for a few minutes afterward. Notice how you feel in your body and in your mind.

- *Bellows breath.* Take a strong breath in and exhale quickly by strongly pumping the abdomen inward. It may be helpful to focus more on the exhale, pushing the breath out with intention, and just letting the breath come back in on its own. Make sure your breath is moving through your nostrils, not the mouth. Your breath should be quite audible, particularly the exhale. It should sound as though air is moving through you with strength. One inhalation and exhalation makes up a cycle; try eight or ten of these at a time. Go slowly at first. You may find this way of breathing more difficult to control; it's not uncommon to find yourself making odd snorting sounds from time to time. Because this is a particularly powerful breath, don't push yourself. Stop if you experience discomfort or dizziness. Lie down and rest for a few minutes afterward, taking the time to register the effect on your body and mind.

Practicing these two exercises with some regularity for a few minutes over the course of several days will give you a taste of the power of the breath. You'll experience for yourself how relaxing and restorative the breath can be when we pay attention to it and work with it. Know that this is only a taste, and that with more extensive practice, under the care of a teacher, you'll have much more striking experiences.

eight

AN OFFICE YOGA ROUTINE

Many of us spend time in offices and end up sitting for hours each day at a desk or computer. When we're at work, we tend to get involved in the task at hand, and we forget about our bodies. We unconsciously get into collapsed, or peculiar, positions, and in a pressured work environment we lose all awareness of our breath. The end result is that our muscles tighten up, our circulation slows down, and our bodies get strained. We get into unhealthy patterns and these become normal—usually until pain wakes us up.

Fortunately, yoga provides ways to cope with—or prevent—these conditions.

It's not that uncommon nowadays to have a yoga class offered at the office. Such classes often take place at lunch and tend to be shorter than regular yoga classes; they're usually only an hour or so. If you have the opportunity to take a lunchtime yoga class, you'll find that it can be a great way to break up your day, give your body some relief, and release some of the stresses of your job. You may even find that taking this time out gives you more energy to continue with your work.

If you don't have the luxury of a noon class, there are several modified yoga postures that you can do on your own. You can do all of these sequentially, or, if you only have time for one or two, then do those. Even a few minutes in these simple positions can help relieve or prevent some of the physical discomforts that often come with office work.

14 SHOULDER ROTATIONS

People who sit at a desk or computer for much of the day often complain of neck and shoulder pain. This pain is a result of the tightening of the muscles in these areas. If left unchecked, neck and shoulder dysfunction can cause pain to radiate down into the arms and fingers. Getting a little movement in the area is the first step toward releasing some of this tension.

Try shrugging your shoulders up toward your ears. Hold this position for a few breaths, and then release your shoulders. Repeat this action a few times, breathing in as you shrug your shoulders up, and breathing out as you release them down. Then try varying the movement by rotating the shoulders in circles. Go several times in each direction, then pause for a moment. Take in how your neck and shoulders feel. You may feel a little more warmth in this general area and you may feel a little looser. This is a good preparatory movement for stretching the neck.

This stretch lengthens the sides of the neck, helping to release tightness and tension in those areas.

Once your neck and shoulders are somewhat loosened by a few shoulder rotations, try tipping your head to one side. Use the hand on the side that you're tilting toward as a light weight. Move into the stretch slowly, only going as far as feels right to

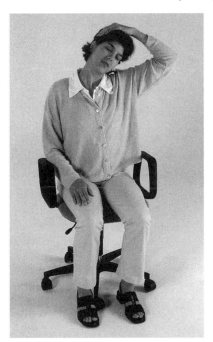

you. Hold this position for a few breaths. To vary it, you can try turning your chin a little more up toward the ceiling or down toward the floor, finding the position that most benefits your neck. Then come back to an upright position. Take a moment before you tip your head over to the other side, repeating the stretch on this side.

Neck Stretch

16 SEATED SPINAL TWIST

This position helps to loosen tightness in the back and neck. It also opens up the chest and creates a light massage of the internal organs as their positions shift.

Sit upright, toward the edge of your chair. Turn toward one side, grasping the side of your leg and the back of the chair if you can reach it. Take a full, slow breath, gently deepening the twist on your exhale. Hold this position for a few breaths, without tensing your body. As a variation, you can try turning your head in the opposite direction of the twist. Release gradually and rest for a breath or two before twisting to the other side.

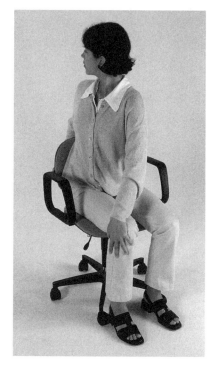

Seated Spinal Twist

This position oxygenates the lungs by opening up the rib cage. It also stretches the arms and shoulders.

Stand facing a wall at a distance that allows you to rest your forehead on the wall. Reach both arms up the wall, above your

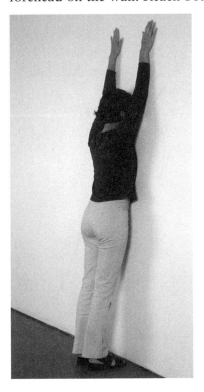

head. If this position pinches your shoulders, you can vary it by widening your arms away from each other until you find the place that feels appropriate. Hold this position for a few breaths, stretching the arms as high as you can.

Wall Stretch

This stretch opens up the chest, reversing the collapsing action that normally occurs with prolonged desk or computer work. It also opens up the shoulders and inner arms.

Stand with one side facing the wall. Reach your arm up the wall, and lean into the wall slightly. You can adjust your distance if you feel too close. Then reach your arm behind you, still along the wall, to about a 45-degree angle, or until you feel a good stretch. If this is too intense for you, step slightly away from the wall, so that the angle of your arm is less extreme. Also, if your arm gets numb or tingly, come out of it and rest for a few breaths.

Hold this position for several breaths. Release out of it slowly, shaking your arm out a little before trying the other side.

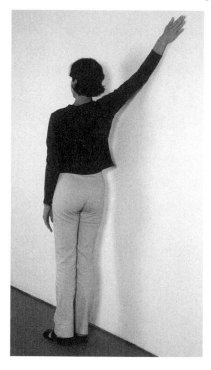

Chest-opening Arm Stretch

TO LEARN MORE

This book gives you a simple introduction to a subject with many other dimensions that are not covered here. The sources listed below will give you a good start if you're interested in reading further. You can also get more information through magazines like *Yoga Journal* and *Yoga International.*

BOOKS

The Art of Sexual Ecstasy, Margo Anand. New York: Tarcher, 1991.
Astanga Yoga: A Practice Guide, Larry Schultz and Janice Gates. (Self-published.)
The Autobiography of a Yogi, Paramahansa Yogananda. Los Angeles: Self-Realization Fellowship, 1981.
Awakening the Spine, Vanda Scaravelli. San Francisco: HarperSan-Francisco, 1995.
The Ayurvedic Cookbook, Amadea Morningstar with Urmila Desai. Twin Lakes, WI: Lotus Light Publications, 1990.
Health, Healing and Beyond: Yoga and the Living Tradition of Krish-namacharya, T. K. V. Desikachar, with R. H. Cravens. New York: Aperture, 1998.

The Heart of Yoga: Developing a Personal Practice, T. K. V. Desikachar. Rochester, VT: Inner Traditions International, 1999.

Light on Yoga, B. K. S. Iyengar. New York: Schocken Books, 1995.

Living with Kundalini, Gopi Krishna. Boston: Shambhala Publications, 1993.

Living Yoga: A Comprehensive Guide for Daily Life, Georg Feuerstein and Stephan Bodian, eds. New York: Tarcher, 1993.

Open Body: Creating Your Own Yoga, Todd Walton. New York: Avon Books, 1998.

Phoenix Rising Yoga Therapy: A Bridge from Body to Soul, Michael Lee. Deerfield Beach, FL: Health Communications, 1997.

Preparing for Birth with Yoga: Exercises for Pregnancy and Childbirth, Janet Balaskas. Boston: Element, 1994.

Relax and Renew: Restful Yoga for Stressful Times, Judith Lasater. Berkeley, CA: Rodmell Press, 1995.)

The Shambhala Guide to Yoga, Georg Feuerstein. Boston: Shambhala Publications, 1996.

The Sivananda Companion to Yoga, Lisa Lidell, et al. New York: Simon and Schuster, 1983.

Tantra: The Path of Ecstasy, Georg Feuerstein. Boston: Shambhala Publications, 1998.

The Tree of Yoga, B. K. S. Iyengar. Boston: Shambhala Publications, 1989.

A Woman's Guide to Tantra Yoga, Vimala McClure. Novato, CA: New World Library, 1997.

Yoga: A Gem for Women, Geeta S. Iyengar. Spokane, WA: Timeless Books, 1991.

Yoga and Ayurveda: Self-Healing and Self-Realization, David Frawley. Twin Lakes, WI: Lotus Light Publications, 1999.

Yoga for Children, Mary Stewart, et al. New York: Fireside, 1993.
Yoga during Pregnancy: Safe and Gentle Stretches, Sandra Jordan. New York: St. Martin's Press, 1988.
Yoga the Iyengar Way, Silva, Mira, and Shyam Mehta. New York: Knopf, 1990.
The Yoga Tradition: Its History, Literature, Philosophy and Practice, Georg Feuerstein. Edmonton, WA: Holm Press, 1998.

VIDEOS

Living Yoga's Abs and Back Care for Beginners, with Rodney Yee
Yoga, Mind, and Body, with Ali MacGraw
Yoga Practice for Beginners, with Patricia Walden
Yoga Practice for Energy, with Rodney Yee
Yoga Practice for Relaxation, with Patricia Walden and Rodney Yee

ACKNOWLEDGMENTS

Many people have contributed to this book. These include all my teachers, as well as the people calling themselves my students. I must also thank the many authors whose books have been so helpful and inspirational to me, especially T. K. V. Desikachar, Georg Feuerstein, and Erich Schiffmann. Thanks to Claudia Schaab at Conari for approaching me about writing this book; thanks are also due to Mary Jane Ryan for her helpful editing. My heartfelt thanks to Rick Fields, who commissioned my articles for *Yoga Journal* and set me on the path of trying to write about self-healing. Many thanks to Liisa O'Maley for making critical last-minute edits and for passing this book around to others to read. I would like to express my gratitude to the Bhansali family—especially Roveen—for being so enthusiastic about my efforts in yoga and for introducing me to India; I also thank my own family, especially my mother, for moral as well as practical support. I'm grateful for the help and support I've received from Julie Staples, Cecile Moochnek, Nancy Friedrich, Jin Sung, Laura Cornell, Todd Jones, and Jonothon Gross.

INDEX

Agitation, *see* rajas

ahimsa, 38–39

Alcott, Bronson (*see also* Transcendentalism), 23

Alexander the Great, 19

Anand, Margot, 85

aparigraha, 38

ardor, *see* tapas

Arjuna (*see also* Bhagavadgita), 19

Art of Sexual Ecstasy, The (*see also* Anand, Margot), 85, 86

asanas (*see also* eight limbs of yoga, asana; postures), 8, 9, 12, 37, 38, 40, 41–42, 43, 50–53, 56, 63, 64, 88, 90, 128, 130, 131

  back bend, 54

  balance poses, 52, 55, 80, 114, 116

  cat stretch/dog tilt, 110–111

  chest-opening arm stretch, 140

child's pose, 112, 113, 114, 124

corpse pose (*see also* shavasana), 12, 13

downward-facing dog, 112–14

floor poses, 52–53

forward bend, 54

handstand, 52

head stand, 52

inverted poses, 52, 84

neck stretch, 137

rocking on the spine, 112, 124–26

seated forward bend, 53, 124, 125, 126

seated spinal twist, 138

shavasana, 12, 13, 54, 62, 83, 90, 98, 128–30

shoulder rotations, 136, 137

shoulder stand, 52

spinal twist, 126–27

148

asanas (*continued*)
    standing forward bend (*see also* uttanasana), 120–21, 126
    standing poses, 51–52, 80, 107
    mountain pose (*see also* tadasana), 116, 120
    tadasana, 114–16
    tree pose, 116–17
    triangle pose, 118–19
    twisting postures, 52–53, 80
    uttanasana, 53, 55, 57, 120–21
    wall stretch, 139
    warrior pose, 88, 122–23
ashram, 77, 79, 80
Ashtanga Vinyasa, *see* Ashtanga yoga
Ashtanga yoga, 25, 72, 75–77
asteya, 38, 39
Atman (*see also* Self), 5
austerity, *see* tapas
Autobiography of a Yogi, The (*see also* Yogananda, Paramahansa), 24, 25, 91
avidya, 32–35, 36
Ayurveda, 66–69

Bandhas, 75
Bhagavadgita, 19, 23
Bhakti yoga, 29
Bikram yoga, 72, 80–81
brahmacharya, 39
breath, breathing (*see also* fire breath; pranayama; ujjayi breath), x, xi, 8, 10, 13, 17, 25, 30, 32, 38, 42, 46, 47, 56–58, 59, 60, 63–64, 75, 79, 80, 90, 96, 103, 109, 131–133, 135
    in poses, 53, 57, 75, 108, 110, 114, 116, 117, 120, 122, 124, 126, 128–29, 136, 137, 138, 139, 140
Buddhism, Buddhist, 17, 19, 36, 39

Celibacy, *see* brahmacharya
Center for Self-Realization (*see also* Yogananda, Paramhansa), 24
chakras, 78–79
chanting, 79–80
Chopra, Deepak, 45
Choudhury, Bikram, 80
Christian, Christianity, 17, 21
clarity, *see* sattva
cleanliness, *see* shaucha

concentration (*see also* eight
  limbs of yoga, dharana), xi, 11,
  38, 46, 56, 86, 114, 116
contentment, *see* santosa
continence, *see* brahmacharya
Desai, Amrit, 81, 82
Desikachar, T. K. V., 25–26, 40,
  46, 47, 91, 101
Devi, Indra, 24
dharana, *see* eight limbs of yoga,
  dharana
dhyana (*see also* eight limbs of
  yoga, dhyana), 38, 42, 43,
  108–109
dreams, 47
duhkha (*see also* suffering), 33,
  35
Ecstasy, 4, 31, 38, 44, 48
eight limbs of yoga (*see also* *Yoga
  Sutras*), 37–44
    asana (*see also* asanas), 38,
      41–42
    dharana, 38, 42, 43
    dhyana (*see also* dhyana), 38,
      42, 43
    niyama, 8, 38, 40–41, 43
    pranayama (*see also*
      pranayama), 38, 42, 43

pratyahara, 38, 42–43
samadhi, 37, 38, 42, 43–44
yama, 8, 37, 38–39, 43
Emerson, Ralph Waldo (*see also*
  Transcendentalism), 23
energy, xi, 6, 9, 11, 36, 39, 52,
  58, 59, 60, 67, 75, 76, 77, 78,
  79, 86, 90, 104, 109, 110, 112,
  122, 124, 135
  centers, *see* chakras
  sealing off, *see* bandhas
  serpentine, *see* kundalini
Feuerstein, Georg, 4, 18, 19,
  20–21, 86
Fields, Rick, 19, 22
fire breath (*see also* Bikram yoga;
  Kundalini yoga), 79, 81
food, xi, 9, 64–66
Gandhi, Mohandas, 30
Ghosh, Bishnu, 80
Greece, 19, 20
gunas, 66–67
guru, 17, 46, 90
Hatha yoga, 8, 17, 21, 29, 30,
  42, 63, 64
Hatha Yoga Pradipika, 30, 64
Health, Healing and Beyond (*see
  also* Desikachar, T. K. V.), 91

Heart of Yoga, The (*see also* Desikachar, T. K. V.), 46
heaviness, *see* tamas
Hinduism, 17
How the Swans Came to the Lake (*see also* Fields, Rick), 46
India, ix, 4, 7, 17, 18, 20, 21, 22, 23, 24, 25, 27, 75, 90–91
ishvara pranidhana (*see also* eight limbs of yoga, niyama), 40, 41
Iyengar, B. K. S., 25, 26, 64, 72–73
Iyengar yoga, 25, 72–74
Jainism, 17
Jnana yoga, 29
Jois, Pattabhi, 25, 75
Jones, Sir William, 21–23
Kabir, 29
Karma yoga, 29
Kripalu yoga, 26, 72, 81–82
Krishna (*see also* *Bhagavadgita*), 19
Krishnamacharya, 24, 25, 40, 75, 101
kundalini, 78, 81
Kundalini yoga, 72, 77–80, 81
Lasater, Judith, 84
Leaves of Grass (*see also* Whitman, Walt), 23

Lee, Michael, 82
life-force, *see* prana
Light on Yoga (*see also* Iyengar, B. K. S.), 64, 73
Mantra yoga, 29, 30
meditation (*see also* dhyana), 30, 38, 44, 61, 108–110, 131
meditation pillow, *see* zafu
Megasthenes, 19
menopause, 100–101
menstrual cycle, 99–100
Mother Teresa, 30
Mirabai, 29
Muir, Charles and Catherine, 85
Niyama, *see* eight limbs of yoga, niyama
non-coveting, *see* aparigraha
non-stealing, *see* asteya
Nusrat Fateh Ali Khan, 29
Obstacles, 8, 46–48
Overeaters Anonymous (*see also* food), 68
Paramahansa, Yoganada, 24, 45, 91
Patanjali, ix, 20, 21
perceiver, *see* purusha
Phoenix Rising Yoga Therapy (*see also* Lee, Michael), 26, 82–83

PMS (premenstrual syndrome), 100

postures (*see also* asanas), ix, x, 3, 8, 9, 10, 11, 17, 38, 41, 42, 50, 51–53, 54, 56, 58, 59, 62, 63, 72, 73, 75, 79, 81, 83, 87, 88, 89, 90, 95, 100, 102, 104, 107, 108, 109, 114, 126, 130, 136

    sequence of (*see also* vinyasa), 53–54, 75, 80, 82, 84, 107, 130, 136

poses, *see* asanas; postures

postpartum yoga, x, 10, 26, 72, 100, 104–105

Power yoga, *see* Ashtanga yoga

prana, 64

pranayama (*see also* breath; eight limbs of yoga, pranayama), 8, 37, 38, 41, 42, 43, 47, 58, 63–64, 90, 128, 130–33

pratyahara, *see* eight limbs of yoga, pratyahara

prenatal yoga, x, 26, 10, 72, 100, 101–104

purity, *see* shaucha

purusha, 5, 35–36

Raja yoga, ix, 29, 30

rajas, 36, 67

Relax and Renew: Restful Yoga for Stressful Times (*see also* Lasater, Judith), 84

relaxation, (*see also* asanas, shavasana), 10, 11, 41, 42, 54, 62–63, 83, 90, 103, 128

restorative yoga, 26, 72, 82, 83–84, 87

restraint, *see* eight limbs of yoga, niyama

Return of the Rishi (*see also* Chopra, Deepak), 45

rishis, 18

Royal Asiatic Society (*see also* Jones, Sir William), 22

"royal road," *see* Raja yoga

Rumi, 22

Samadhi, *see* eight limbs of yoga, samadhi

Sanskrit, 4, 22, 33

santosa (*see also* eight limbs of yoga, niyama), 40

sattva, 36, 67

satya, 38, 39

Scaravelli, Vanda, 87

seer, *see* rishis

Self (*see also* svadhyaya), 5, 14, 32, 41, 44, 98

self-realization, 5, 8, 29, 37

sense withdrawal, *see* eight limbs
of yoga, pratyahara
serpentine energy, *see* kundalini
shaucha (*see also* eight limbs of
yoga, niyama), 40
shavasana, *see* asanas, shavasana
Shri Aurobindo, 18
siddhis, 44–46
Sikh, Sikhism, 17, 77–78, 80
Stewart, Mary, 87
suffering (*see also* duhkha), 1, 4,
33, 35
svadhyaya (*see also* eight limbs of
yoga, niyama), 40, 41
Swami Vivekananda, ix, 24
Tadasana, *see* asanas, tadasana
tamas, 36, 66, 67
Tantra yoga, 21, 72, 85–86
Tantra: The Path of Ecstasy (*see
also* Feuerstein, Georg), 86
tapas (*see also* eight limbs of
yoga, niyama), 40–41
Thoreau, Henry David (*see also*
Transcendentalism), 23
T.M. (transcendental meditation),
30
Transcendentalism, 23
truth telling, *see* satya

Ujjayi breath (*see also* Ashtanga
yoga; Bikram yoga), 57–58, 75,
80–81, 132
Upanishads, 18, 19
uttanasana, *see* asanas, uttanasana
Vedas, 18
Vedic tradition, 66
vegetarianism, vegetarian (*see
also* food), 23, 65–66, 78
vinyasa, 54, 75, 76
Wheels of the body, *see* chakras
Whitman, Walt (*see also* Transcendentalism), 23
World Parliament of Religions,
23
Yama, *see* eight limbs of yoga,
yama
yoga
and emotional release, 82–83
and food, *see* food
and menopause, *see*
menopause
and menstruation, *see* menstrual cycle, 100
and sex, *see* Tantra yoga
at the office, 135–40
audiotapes, 97

devotional, *see* Bhakti yoga

for children, 86–87

for the disabled, 88–89

for the elderly, 87–88

for postpartum women, *see* postpartum yoga

for pregnant women, *see* prenatal yoga

for women, 99–105

history of, 3–4, 7, 17–25, 45, 72, 75, 77, 80

meaning of the Sanskrit word, 4, 62

of everything, *see* Tantra yoga

of force, *see* Hatha yoga

of selfless action, see Karma yoga

of wisdom, *see* Jnana yoga

props (*see also* Iyengar yoga; prenatal yoga; restorative yoga), 73–74, 84, 87, 96–97, 102

teachers, 3, 46, 50, 71, 72, 79, 80, 84, 85, 87, 89–96, 98, 101, 104, 133

videos, 89, 90, 97

Yoga College of India (*see also* Choudhury, Bikram), 80

Yoga Flow, 26, 72

Yoga for Children (*see also* Stewart, Mary), 87

Yoga Movement, 26, 72

Yogananda, Paramahansa, 24, 80

Yoga Rahasaya, 101

Yoga Sutras (*see also* Patanjali), 20, 30, 31–32, 33–34, 36, 37, 44, 46, 47, 58

Yoga Tradition, The (*see also* Feuerstein, Georg), 18, 20

Yogi Bhajan, 77

yogis, 3, 18, 24, 25, 44–45

special powers of, *see* siddhis

Zafu, 108, 131

ABOUT THE AUTHOR

Cybèle Tomlinson is the Director of the Berkeley Yoga Center. A longtime yoga teacher and bodyworker, she also writes for *Yoga Journal*. She lives in Berkeley, California.

A Simple Wisdom Book

Simple Yoga is part of Conari Press' A Simple Wisdom Book series which seeks to provide accessible books on enlightening topics.

Other titles in the Simple Wisdom Book series:

Simple Meditation & Relaxation
by Joel Levey and Michelle Levey

Simple Feng Shui by Damian Sharp

Simple Kabbalah by Kim Zetter

Simple Chinese Astrology by Damian Sharp

CONARI PRESS

2550 Ninth Street, Suite 101
Berkeley, California 94710-2551
800-685-9595   510-649-7175
fax: 510-649-7190   e-mail: conari@conari.com
www.conari.com